'Full of wisdom and delight and will be a great inspiration to anyone who has felt lost or stranded'
Amy Liptrot – Bestselling author of *The Outrun*

'Inspiring, funny and touching – often on the same page'
Rachael Lucas

'It's real, it's raw and it's hopeful'
Lisa Bradley

'A wonderful blend of humour and honest grief – I read the whole thing in a sitting'
Miriam Landor

'Moving, witty and wise – I alternately cheered and teared up through her inspiring and transformative year'
Shauna Reid

'I absolutely loved it! – it is so relatable, I cried quite a few times and cheered Sarah on as she found joy in wild swims'
Lisa Irwin

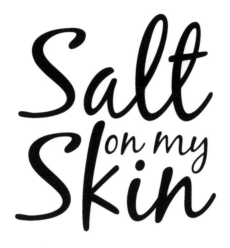

Salt on my Skin

Sarah Kennedy Norquoy

Published in 2020 by Welford Publishing
Copyright © Sarah Kennedy Norquoy 2020

ISBN: 978-1-9162671-3-8

Book mentor Cassandra Farren
Front cover image © Jessica Barnes
Front cover design © Jen Parker, Fuzzy Flamingo
Author photograph © Dave Rendall
Editor Christine McPherson

A catalogue for this book is available from the British Library.

To my younger self.

You had no idea how strong you were.

Disclaimer

This book is designed to provide helpful information on the subjects discussed. It is general reference information which should not be used to diagnose any medical problem and is not intended as a substitute for consulting with a medical or professional practitioner.

Wild swimming is a wonderful and fun activity, but readers should be aware that it comes with risk. Everyone is advised to research fully the dangers of wild swimming before embarking on this activity and do so at their own risk. Salt On My Skin is the author's personal journey and not a guide.

Some names and identifying details have been changed to protect the privacy of the individuals.

Red braids and self-loathing

'm not your most obvious choice of woman to be writing a book about sea swimming. In fact, I'm not an obvious choice to be writing about swimming at all. As a child, I was the last person to learn to swim in my class, and the whole thing was misery. Our primary school had an outdoor pool, and in the summer we took our lessons there. That was my first experience of outdoor swimming – and I hated it. First, because I couldn't swim; and second, my clearest memory of it was how cold the water was. It was 'allegedly' a heated pool, but it was forever out of use waiting for the maintenance man to come and fix the heater. Truth is, he probably couldn't even find the blessed heater because there was NO HEAT!

Swimming achievements at the school were awarded through a poor man's badge of honour system. When you could swim a width, you were awarded a small piece of red braid which your mother dutifully sewed onto your swimming costume. Then, when you swam a length, you were given your blue braid. Jumping in, sitting on the side to dive in, collecting a weighted stick from the bottom, and swimming in your pyjamas (why?) all earned you a different coloured piece of braid, which the alpha kids wore on their swimsuits like medals.

I struggled to get my first braid, and my swimsuit stayed naked for what felt like years. The humiliation was tough.

One summer, the teacher must have taken pity on both me and the one other pupil – a boy – who hadn't achieved anything in the lab-rat braiding system, and she told us to be at school for 8am one Wednesday in the summer term. This was unheard of; it was the seventies! In those days, there was no person-centred support for learning at all; we just piled into the class and either achieved or didn't. So, for the teacher to ask us to get to school early to swim a width and get our red braid was monumental.

I don't recall her name, but I can still see her silhouette of wavy dark hair and bad seventies trouser suit as she screamed, 'COME ON, COME ON, COME ON!' to me as I energetically doggie-paddled my way across the pool. I vividly recall myself doing it, determined not to touch the bottom and lose out on my one and only chance to get the 4-inch piece of red braid. I ran home, bursting with excitement as I proudly showed off my award, which was cut straight across the top for hemming and sewing on, and kite-tailed at the bottom to prevent fraying. I think there are still photos of me in a swimsuit with the red braid sewn onto it. Finally, I could swim a width. I had a red braid. I could do hard things.

I have no recollection of collecting any more braids.

I probably did, but they just didn't have the same value as that first one. I'm pretty certain I never swam in my pyjamas, though, and I've never understood why that was a requirement. If in adult life you go trooping down the water's edge in your nightie, it would look a bit weird and people would start asking questions about your sanity. If you did it as a child, your parents would be questioned as to the level of your care.

Once I'd mastered the basics, I went on to swim with the classes on a regular basis. In the pool we were required to wear those monstrous swimming hats that barely fitted over your head, ripped patches of hair out of your scalp on removal, gave you a massive headache, pushed your eyes down to your chin, and were covered in gaudy flowers. The youth of today have no idea how easy they have it. No hideous, head-squashing swim hat? No swim. Suck it up.

★

At periods throughout my adult life, I have swum on and off in reasonably regular bursts. When I was pregnant with my second child, the clocks had gone back and I decided to be productive with my extra hour, so I went swimming in the local pool. I loved it so much I went three or four times a week throughout the entire pregnancy. I was fitter than I'd been in a long time, had a super easy labour, and lost a stone in pregnancy. Twelve weeks later, my husband left me.

Suddenly, I was a single parent to my six-year-old daughter Katie and my new-born son Elliot, and I don't think I entered the water again properly for nearly ten years. I would go through phases of swimming regularly, but by then I'd gained weight and the hardest part was the walk of shame from the changing room to the pool. I hated myself, and there's only so much sucking in that it's humanly possible to do without passing out. Reader, you do NOT want to pass out in a swimsuit. Imagine having to be rescued in that compromising position. Quite frankly, I'd rather you left me there to die.

It turns out that tall, skinny friends are equally hung up about their bodies. We are all comparing and wishing we had more of the other person, who is simultaneously wishing they had less of themselves. This is what creates the multi-million pound business which makes people pay money to go to classes and be told they are overweight (over what weight exactly?) when they can achieve that by just looking in the mirror for free. I am one of those people. I'm not proud of it, but I have a loathing of my body which I've been nurturing for upwards of thirty years. I go through phases when I don't mind myself so much. But on the whole, if someone goes to take my photograph, I'm usually barking orders for them to hold the camera up, get my chins out, get someone to stand in front of me, hide my stomach, legs, arms, chest... My face is ok, but from the neck down I'd rather you didn't go there.

It's worth saying something at this point, before you

dive further into the book. You may come across times throughout the chapters where I make references or jokes about my body which make you twitch. If you're body positive, or are happy with your body and have done the mindset and emotional work, then I applaud you. If you're comfortable with what you see in the mirror without external validation, then that's excellent. If you're struggling like I do, then I hear you. This book is the story of the journey I am on, and reflects how I felt at the time. I'm slowly improving, but progress is often two steps forward and one back. Sometimes we run, sometimes we walk, sometimes we sit down and don't move for a long time. I'm travelling along the same road; we are all just in different places on it.

So, have I set the scene as to why I'm a highly unlikely candidate to be writing about sea swimming when there is no hiding and no escape? Why is this woman – publicly the last to learn to swim and hates being seen in anything other than a big heavy coat which hides all – not only hopping into the sea at every opportunity and dressing by the side of the car in all weathers, but also writing about it?

It's because, against all the odds, sea swimming saved me in 2019, and a transformation has taken place. I found my thing, and I hope to inspire you to find yours.

Sink or Swim

couldn't stop crying. The pain in my heart was so bad it was almost physical, and there felt like a perpetual round of tears that I was set to drown in. I was devastated, utterly heartbroken, and once again having to dig deep and pull up all the resources I needed to stay strong after what felt like a lifetime of doing just that. My usual buoyant sense of humour and Pollyanna can-do attitude had flatlined. I wanted to crawl into a cave and sleep for five years. I was distraught.

It was January 31st, 2019, and I was sitting sobbing in my car at what was already shaping up to be the worst year ever – and we were only one month in. One of my closest friends, Fiona, had died of cancer less than two weeks into January, and the loss of her sat heavy on my heart.

When I made the monumental move from Cambridge to Orkney some 11 years previously, she'd been my rock and cheerleader and had even put out flags in the garden for my arrival, making me feel so included and valued. And now she was gone, forever.

We'd shared a million memories and the same quirky sense of humour, the same love of lighthouses and rainbows, and hours and hours in each other's company. When we had to transport a rolled-up carpet down a hill in the snow, it was no problem. She simply strapped it to the top of a Ford Fiesta and drove down with it on the roof, styling it out wonderfully whilst I was a nervous wreck. 'Fiestas stick to the roads like glue,' she cheerfully informed me. I hear her say that so often whilst I'm driving in challenging conditions now, even though I no longer even have a Fiesta. If Fiona can drive down a hill in the snow with a carpet strapped to the roof, then surely it was a lesson that I needed to stop saying 'I can't', and start saying 'I can'.

This is just one of many memories that fill me with such joy; she threw her heart and soul into everything with great gusto. Following her diagnosis, she had continued to stay resilient which put me and all around her to shame. Even when she stayed in Macmillan, I visited her with a friend who had taken a gin and tonic in a gift bag for Fiona to look forward to when she got home again. Instead, she tipped her glass of water back in the jug, poured the G&T into the glass and swallowed her painkillers, reassuring the nurse that yes she had something to take them with and held up her glass full of contraband liquid! My friend and I stared in total silence and horror, dreading being caught like naughty schoolgirls.

No-one did Fiona like Fiona. She really was one in a million… and now she was gone. Why does life have to be so cruel? It felt like so much had died along with her. The secret jokes only we understood, the hours and hours of MSN messages we had shared, whacky adventures taken, text messages, and the knowledge that there was someone who always had my back. It was all gone. I'd sobbed wretchedly at her funeral when her coffin was put into the hearse to be driven away, my crying so loud that Fiona's husband came over to comfort me.

Now I was crying again. This time, I was alone in my car, and my grief was for the loss of someone who was still living – my mother. At that moment, I felt totally wretched and desperately alone.

An image from minutes earlier was etched before me and will stay with me forever. It was of my parents standing in the snow outside the hospital, huddled together whilst my mum was crying. Interspersed between the sobs, we stared like rabbits caught in the headlights of a car. Mum looked up from Dad's shoulder and said, with that now all too familiar bewildered face, 'What have I been diagnosed with again?'

'It's vascular dementia, Mum.'

In the five minutes it had taken her to walk up the corridor and out into the harsh January air, she had already forgotten her devastating diagnosis.

My parents have endured an awful lot in their many years together: Dad had survived a quadruple bypass; Mum had survived breast and colon cancer; and together their hearts were broken with the loss of their son to suicide.

Seeing them so frightened and vulnerable once again

was almost too much for me to bear. I had to leave them to drive back home, both terrified of what was to come but trying to be brave. Meanwhile, I had to get my own brave on and return to work with a face that had quickly reached the ugly crying stage.

There was only one tiny chink of light in what looked set to be a horrible indefinite time ahead. Thanks to a midlife crisis a few weeks before, I'd taken to sea swimming.

As I sat staring down the lens of 50, I'd set myself a list of 49 new experiences for the year leading up to it, in a completely unachievable, setting myself up to fail, bucket list. I was already so busy I frequently met myself coming back the other way. I was permanently stressed out of my box, newly grieving for my friend, and had spent the last year looking for a diagnosis for my mother. So, what the heck, why not throw sea swimming in January into the heady mix?

Yet somehow, I'd tried it two weeks earlier and taken to it straight away. And before I knew it, sea swimming had become a thing.

I was set to cry a lot of salty tears in the coming months. But I had absolutely no comprehension of how sea swimming and a different kind of salt on my skin was going to save me.

January 2019, the nightmare of all years. It was sink or swim.

I chose to swim.

January

'A sunset swim in the sea, in the last light of the day, with company at first then they left the water and I was alone with just a solitary seal watching from a distance. Something incredible is happening to me. I only started sea swimming nine days ago. I'm overwhelmed.'

(Diary entry)

've always been a huge fan of the ocean. Growing up in the land-locked Midlands, the sea was a great source of mystery and excitement because I only ever saw it for my two weeks' holiday. We'd be packed off in the car, three of us squashed in the back with all our holiday clap-trap piled around us, and our only entertainment being a list of things to spot on the journey as we drove the miles and miles to the coast. A blue car, a telephone box, a lady in a red coat, a castle, and so on. The final thing on the list was always 'the sea'. And I feel emotional even as I write this, because it always filled me with such excitement to finally see it. I felt as though I had reached the end of the earth; I could paddle and splash and listen to the waves… something I have never tired of for as long as my memory tells me.

I've always been a dreamer and the sea really lends itself to that, as it hosts a million untold stories and legends. When I was younger, I longed for mermaids to be real. When I moved to Orkney, I joined a local church, and it was here I met and later married a local fisherman called Roy – often nicknamed by me as Orkney Beef. Fishermen have many stories from their time at sea, and he once told the children that just because we had never seen a mermaid didn't mean they weren't real. This has stuck with him, and he is teased about it many times, but I love these myths and legends. To this very day, I believe I saw a sea horse whilst playing in the shallow waves as a little girl. That hope of a little magic out there has never left me.

My move from Cambridge to Orkney 11 years ago had been for a number of reasons. Mainly it was a 'call' I couldn't ignore. The 'call' had gone on for a number of years, and I'd been to visit alone while my parents looked after my children back in Cambridge. I knew it was somewhere I wanted to live but wasn't prepared to risk everything and chuck in a happy life in Cambridge on a gamble. So, I placed it on the back burner for years, with the acceptance that what was for me would not go by me and I could always revisit the idea again in the future.

A mutual friend had put me in touch with Fiona and we quickly connected. When she told me about an event coming up called 'Islands Ablaze', I knew I wanted to go. It was a joint church event over a few days, and Fiona invited me to stay in her home while I attended. That visit cemented my desire to move, and Fiona helped me to find somewhere to live. From the outside looking in, I can see people shaking their heads and saying it was a HUGE gamble – and it was. But it was one I felt ready to make some four years after my initial visit, and everything fell into place.

Just a few weeks prior to my moving, Mum became very ill with a rare and severe form of bowel cancer. She was taken into hospital to have the tumour and a large part of her colon removed, and as Dad and I travelled to visit her I told him that I would call the plans off and not move. I would stay close to them. I vividly remember that Mum was recovering from her operation, with oxygen tubes in her nose and lines in her arms for fluid and antibiotics.

Dad, who was sitting next to her bed, leaned in and said, 'Sarah's talking about not going to Orkney now.'

Mum could barely lift her head off the pillow, but she turned and looked at me and said firmly, 'You're going.' And that was that.

I might argue from time to time with God about what I should be doing and where I should be going, but I daren't argue with *The Mothership* as she's been fondly known as for many years. So, I obeyed orders and went.

Mum made a full and miraculous recovery, and she and Dad followed me to Orkney a year later, following the tragic death of my brother Simon. My sister Ann had been living in Colorado for many years, Simon had lived in Florida, and now I was in Orkney. It seemed an obvious choice to move to close to one of us, and they have never regretted the move to these special islands.

Despite the difficulties and sadness of leaving behind friends, family, and people I loved, somewhere high up on the list of my reasons to move was to finally live by the sea. The first house I moved into had a view of the sea from my front room, and I simply couldn't believe my luck. I moved house a few times as I found somewhere to settle, but each home had a sea view. Fiona, the friend who had made me feel so welcome, had even let me live in her home while she was abroad, and she had a balcony that opened out to a sea view.

My home now looks down onto the Bay of Skaill, which hosts the ancient Neolithic settlement Skara Brae.

Living on an island, not a day goes by where I don't see the sea. If I want to calm myself down, think to the end of my thought, dream, or reset, then the sea is the place to go. Beaches are full of negative ions which increase the flow of oxygen to the brain, improving mood and reducing stress. Sometimes on my way home from work, I just pull into the parking spot that looks out to the sea just below my home. On wild and windy days, I've been known to jump in my car, head down there, and just watch. Just be. Just sea.

Despite a lifetime love of the sea and being surrounded by it for the past ten years, I'd had no desire to swim in it at all since moving to Orkney. My childhood fearlessness had long since left and adult mindset well and truly kicked in. 'It looks far too cold,' I told myself a million times, thus sealing my decision to enjoy it from a safe splashing distance.

Sitting in the car waiting for the others to arrive for my first sea swim was the most nervous I'd been in a long time. I also felt a bit ridiculous. Me, an overweight woman in a borrowed wetsuit, about to head into the icy cold waters in January, when there was no guarantee I wouldn't make a complete spectacle of myself and hyperventilate, freak out, and need assistance... or perhaps die! I'd even casually asked prior to the event if a doctor would be present. No-one was forcing my hand, but once I'd committed to doing it, this was something I had to go through with. As I anxiously waited, I reflected on how I'd got to this stage.

Less than a month earlier, I'd just entered my 50th year. As mentioned earlier, I'd celebrated my final year in my forties by compiling a challenge of 49 new experiences. Some of these were small things, like try a new food or drink; some were bigger things, like ride a camel (#pray4camel), ride in a submarine, see a calf being born, and learn how to play the piano. Wild swimming – or a polar bear dip, as I'd named it – also went on the list. When people ask me how and why I started sea swimming in January, I tell them it was my midlife crisis bucket list. It seems there are no limits to what a perimenopausal woman is capable of.

I was aware of a small group of people who regularly

swam in the sea in Orkney, and a friend of mine was always telling me how good she felt afterwards. I would listen and smile, but in my head I always filed it under the 'never' category. So, I don't know how never became maybe, but at some point it crossed over, and I found myself joining the Facebook group and voicing an intention to give it a try. I was inundated with messages of encouragement, although most people suggested leaving it until the summer.

However, a few days later, a stranger – now friend – Alette, turned up at my workplace with a wet suit, gloves, and shoes, and started speaking about, 'When we go on Saturday...'.

Wait...

WHAT?

Saturday as in three days away in January, not Saturday as in six months away in the summer?

A combination of shame and determination found me nodding in agreement to the planned swim, and I was to go home and somehow squash myself into the wetsuit and get my backside down to the beach on Saturday morning.

The nerves kicked in virtually straight away, but despite this I was also a tiny bit excited. So, that evening I tried on my borrowed wetsuit for size. I didn't bother to put a swimsuit on, but just tried it on over my underwear. The struggle was real, and I went through to the sitting room and told my husband I was having a bit of difficulty 'getting it all in', as I couldn't zip it up. After he put his eyes back in his head, he told me I had it on back to front and I'd have a much easier job putting the zip to the back. Ah…

Saturday arrived, and it was pretty windy. Not long before the swim was due, I'd received a message from Alette saying the more experienced Polar Bears had felt it wasn't a good idea to take a newbie to the proposed beach, because it wasn't sheltered and my first go would be miserable. After psyching myself for days, I couldn't believe how disappointed I was that the swim was now called off, which showed I was ready. Thankfully, Alette was determined to get me in the water, and quickly sourced another swim spot that would be much more protected from the wind.

During the war, a series of causeways were constructed to connect the south isles to the mainland of Orkney and to prevent warships getting through. Several shipwrecks lie here, and it's a popular place for divers to come and explore. Known as the Churchill Barriers, we refer to them as Barrier One, Two, Three, and Four.

Barrier One was the chosen place, with the beautiful Italian chapel built by Italian prisoners of war as the backdrop. What an exquisite place to start. It was also about a 25-minute drive from my home, and I'd been advised to drive in my wetsuit to save me trying to put it on when there. The sight of me getting into the darn thing in public could have led to rescue teams trying to harpoon me and drag me back in the water, so I didn't need telling twice!

I'd arrived early, so sat in the car looking out at the water, and was almost moved to tears to see a vibrant rainbow right over the place we were going to swim. Rainbows are incredibly special to me, so when I see them at times of significance, I always feel like it's God telling me it's going to be ok. Call me dramatic, but I took this as a sign that God was telling me I wouldn't die or, at the very least, need rescuing like some beached whale. Oh, dear Lord, here come the nerves again…

The others arrived and we made our way down to the beach, across the stones from the car park, and put our things a little way from the water's edge. I still recall so much about that first swim. I can picture myself standing at the water's edge and walking in. Alette was calmly talking to me and encouraging me as I waded in; I was so pumped by this stage, I don't think I even felt the cold. She told me I could get out at any point, I didn't have to put my shoulders under, and I could come back another day. But I hadn't come this far to only come this far.

So, before Alette was even in the water herself, I was fully submerged, shoulders in, and away off swimming! I remember shouting, 'I CAN DO HARD THINGS!' as I swam. It's my favourite phrase and mantra which I say daily to myself and often to other people. I felt absolutely euphoric, and so the love affair began.

Fiona had been excited to see me working my way through my list of 49 things, and had asked me to show photos along the way. So, as I quickly dressed after my swim and journeyed home, I decided to stop off at hers to show her. By then, Fiona's cancer was quickly taking over and we knew she didn't have long left. I let myself into her house and saw her sitting in a chair with oxygen, and I knew this would be the last time I saw her this side of heaven.

When I showed her the photos, she spoke quietly – speaking being an effort – and we shared a special hour together. I have so many memories of my beautiful, fun friend, and as I reflect on that last hour spent with her, I remain so thankful for the unchanging and unconditional love and support she showed to me on my arrival to Orkney.

Fiona was becoming tired, signalling it was time for me to leave. I couldn't bring myself to say goodbye in any official way, but as I stood up to go, she put her hand out to me and we held hands for a moment without a word. I knew. She knew. I leaned down, kissed the top of her head, and said, 'Thank you for all the fun.' I left in tears.

Those were the first tears of many I was going to shed that year.

Fiona died peacefully the following day. I would never see her again. She was gone, leaving a huge hole in my life. And even now, as I write almost a year later, I still can't quite believe she's not here. I often popped in a few times a week for a quick hello, but I doubt I would have gone that particular Saturday if it wasn't to show her my photos to prove I had done it, mainly because

I didn't want to get in the way knowing a lot of people wanted to see her in the last days.

Sea swimming made that final visit happen. The timing had been perfect, and I will always be thankful for that beautiful arrangement of time.

★

As I dressed hurriedly on the beach from my very first swim, a lady turned to me saying, 'I'll warn you, it's very addictive.' I had loved my first sea swim, but I couldn't imagine it becoming addictive.

I'd gone home feeling exhilarated and incredibly proud of myself for doing the hard thing, and I certainly knew I wanted to do it again. I guess addiction is something that develops and doesn't happen instantly. But now I would say yes, I am addicted. Within a matter of a few short swims, I found myself viewing my beloved sea in a completely different way. I scanned the water the whole time, looking at the tides, the sea state, if there was a place to get in easily, and, more importantly, get out easily. Rule number one of swimming: before you enter the water, make sure you can exit it as well. I have known river swimmers to take a ladder to enable them to get out of the water.

I was drawn to water like a magnet: no longer for gazing at, but to be fully immersed in it. I knew nothing of the science behind what happens when you enter the cold water. I simply knew that I had to do it as often as I could.

I began to share my experiences through my online blog, and realised that the small community of people I thought did this was actually a much bigger one. If I wasn't swimming outdoors, I was dreaming about swimming outdoors, reading about swimming outdoors, or looking at pictures of other people swimming outdoors. Addiction may not have taken hold, but by this stage I was certainly hooked.

My fourth swim had been splashy. I'd swum with a friend or rather '*had a knockabout in the sea*' as she worded it. Not really swimming weather, it had been great for having a good splash about in the cold, settling our emotions, and getting a face full of waves in the process. We hurried home and dressed quickly, ready to sit by the fire with hot drinks to warm up.

I brushed my cheek and felt the lovely sensation of dried salt on my cheeks, eyebrows, even my lashes. And at that moment, a secondary addiction was born. The feeling of salt on my skin and smoothing it away is my guilty pleasure. You heard it here first.

In the beginning, I was wearing a wetsuit all the time, but was full of admiration for those who swam 'skins'. This means swimming in just your swimsuit, and is not to be mistaken for skinny dipping! Many people said it was far more preferable.

The majority of swimmers had a big, heavy, post-swim coat/changing robe. There are many to choose from on the market, and I was advised from day one that I would be better to invest in a change-robe than a wetsuit. This turned out to be a superb piece of advice, and I feel like I live in my change robe. Other, more experienced swimmers were pretty convinced I'd be in skins eventually, and explained that most people who'd bought a wetsuit had quickly discarded it.

I was not so convinced about skins, but decided I needed to at least give it a try. There were lots of tips for going from wetsuit to skins. Some people take their wetsuit off in the water at the end of a swim, so they have a few seconds or a minute or two to begin to acclimatise. I decided to just try skins one morning, thinking, *If they can do it, so can I.* After all, I can do hard things!

It was the morning of Fiona's funeral, and there was a planned swim at a beach called Inganess. This has now become one of my most frequent places to swim but, amazingly, even after ten years in Orkney, I had never been there prior to that day. What makes Inganess so distinctive is the shipwreck that sits close to the shore in the bay. Called the *Juniata*, it was an old block ship built in 1918. It had originally sunk in around 1940, near Barrier Four, then reclaimed and taken to Inganess Bay to be broken up. But after 80 years, it's never been touched, and probably never will. It's now rusty, covered in mussels, and incredibly atmospheric.

That morning was another cold and frosty one, crisp and clear. My husband and parents would be going to Fiona's funeral in the afternoon, and I had taken the day off work to attend. I'd had a variety of jobs since arriving in Orkney. Working in a restaurant, a flower shop (which happened to be the coldest and loveliest job I've known), a library, and as a home carer. Now I was a support worker, which suited me like a hand in a glove, and provided me with a secure contract and fortunately a degree of flexibility.

I thought on the day of the funeral that a good way to distract myself for the morning would be to go along to the swim and try going in with just Lycra leggings and a t-shirt. It wasn't skins, but it certainly wasn't a wetsuit.

The difference in the feel was remarkable. As I walked into the sea, I can remember thinking the cold was intolerable and there was no way I'd stay in longer than a couple of minutes. I began to hyperventilate and had to force myself to breathe slowly. *Do your labour breathing*, I reminded myself, but was on the edge of beginning to panic. I stayed within my depth – something I always do if swimming alone – and shouted to the others that I would only be a few minutes as it was so cold. But remarkably, after a couple of minutes I began to adjust.

After the initial violence of really uncomfortable cold, I found I had acclimatised and was able to swim for 15 minutes. The water was crystal clear and there was hardly a ripple. For some reason, this swim is fixed very clearly in my mind, and I wonder if it's because I connect it to Fiona's funeral day or because it was my first time without a wetsuit, or both. But whatever it was, this swim ended up being very clearly a memorable and special one.

As always, we dressed quickly and made for our

hot drinks. Hands unable to function due to cold, teeth chattering, and frosty breath, yet all exhilarated and ready for the warm glow that starts within a few minutes of exiting the water.

As much as that swim was memorable, I found my recovery took much longer without a wetsuit. So, I decided I wasn't ready to give it up just yet, and returned to wearing it for the next few swims.

It's normal for me to really struggle in January. Christmas is back in its box, and we are all plunged back into darkness as the festive lights are taken down, or at the very least switched off. This is when people like me (whingers) have to dig deep to make it through to spring.

I often have a massive falling-out with Orkney at this time of year and talk about moving, usually during another great January storm. Orkney is a beautiful place to live, but even with all it has to offer, I find it difficult in January and February because it's still so dark and hard going. One of the things which keeps me going in January is the first snowdrop sighting. My favourite and most poignant of flowers always heralds the end of winter, and is a sign that hope is just around the corner. New life is bursting through. The misery will soon be over. We can make it to spring; we can do it. Snowdrops have saved me many times.

As we crept on through wintry days, I found myself beginning to see a slight change in my attitude towards life outside during winter. After spending a lifetime of winters dashing from the house to the car and the car to work, I was now beginning to spend more time outdoors – and strangely not hating it.

I use various forms of social media, and one year I bemoaned winter on Twitter, not being backwards in coming forwards about how much I hated it. I remember Amy Liptrot (author of the spectacular book, *The Outrun*) encouraging me to try and embrace the elements of winter instead of hating it. I knew she was right, but I just couldn't bring myself to.

One February, I was off work sick. The weather was monstrous, and I sat by the fire reading *The Outrun* from cover to cover. Amy lived and grew up only a couple of miles from where I live, and we share roughly the same view. Her book, her love of Orkney, and her descriptions, made me fall back in love with the islands again, and gave me the strength I needed to get through the last weeks of that winter. No easy feat!

But since starting sea swimming, I was now finding it easier, and taking in so many of the wonderful colours that I usually missed. The skies, clouds, fields, horizons, and landscape, were all a glorious mix of dark brooding clouds, yellow to pink sunsets, and every conceivable colour of blue, green, and turquoise in the sea. I marvelled at how the landscape changed twice a day with the changing tide, bringing in new treasures from the ocean, washing away the memories of the previous twelve hours. Instead of moaning about the perpetual mud, I was seeing beyond to the sunlight bursting through dark clouds.

Orkney has its own language, with many words, phrases and meanings never heard elsewhere. 'Solja' means the brilliant sunshine between showers, and describes it beautifully.

Solja. Brilliant sunshine between showers. I am absolutely here for it.

As much as I was falling in love with a new hobby, though, there were difficulties with my mum. As yet, she was undiagnosed, and this was proving a constant source of anxiety. I had begun to see changes in the previous year. In fact, in the January the year before, I remember meeting her in the library, which was a favourite place for both of us. As we stood speaking in the entrance, I commented on how anxious she was becoming and wondered if it would be a good idea for her to go to the doctor.

I had no idea what was going to unfold, and at the time, no expectation whatsoever of the diagnosis she would receive just 12 months later. But I guess for me it was the first time I had noticed there were tiny cracks appearing in my strong and capable mum, 'The Mothership'. Tiny cracks where, instead of light shining through, something else was leaking out. Anxiety, repetition of questions, forgetfulness, and sometimes an inability to do a very simple task.

I remember with a heavy heart one Sunday around this time when she was sitting at our dinner table and I noticed that her hearing aid was sitting strangely in her ear, so I pointed it out. She took the hearing aid out and began to fiddle with it. I cannot to this day describe what the uneasy feeling was in me that makes me recall this very minor incident, but she just fiddled with it, and neither fixed it nor put it back in her ear. To my shame, I remember becoming impatient with her, and I snatched it out of her hand, corrected it, and put it back in her ear.

I still hate myself for that ten seconds of impatience I showed, because I can never go back and change it. It sits there in history now and forever more. After being raised and fed and nurtured and loved by my mother as I grew from baby to toddler, finding my way and making mistakes, that day I didn't show her the grace she needed or help her like she had helped me.

It was just one of those moments that has stuck with me. In my mind, it's probably bigger than the event. And as I often say to Dad when he has a moment, 'The moment doesn't define the marriage.' I've since apologised to Mum, but she had no recollection of it, proving it sits heavier on my heart than it does hers. My few seconds over a hearing aid doesn't define the relationship I have with my mum. It's just one of many times where, if I had the opportunity to go back, I'd have done it differently.

As 2018 progressed, the tiny cracks and leaks became bigger and bigger. My husband and I went to my parents' house for dinner one evening – something fairly routine – and Mum was wandering around the kitchen in a complete daze, unable to process and function. It was the first time I knew something was really wrong. She was utterly bewildered, and when I went home that night I made a doctor's appointment myself, told my parents when it was happening, and that I would be going with them.

Mum had been put on some anti-anxiety tablets a couple of months before, and we questioned if these might be affecting her. But I had a gut feeling it was something more than that, and had to tread carefully.

She dutifully attended various appointments, all the time protesting that she was absolutely fine and only there to reassure me that she wasn't going mad. But I continued to have my concerns, and the appointments to rule out certain things had all been exhausted. It all led to a psychiatrist appointment in January 2019, which resulted in me crying my eyes out in the car. A life-changing hour, sitting in the hospital room answering question after question. Sometimes they were aimed directly at Mum, sometimes at me or Dad, but all resulting in a dementia diagnosis that was going to shatter us. Right there and then, the future looked cold and bleak, and there was not a solitary snowdrop in sight.

February

Last night I dreamed about Mum and she was young and ok. I awoke grief-stricken, there were tears on my pillow. I was thankful for a day off so went down to the sea close to home. It's possible to cry and swim at the same time, I've discovered. Salty tears merge with the sea and both heal me.

(Diary entry)

I hate winter and always have. February is always the hardest month for me to endure because we've been doing winter for quite some time by then, and there's no sign of it abating any time soon. Spring feels a million miles away, and renewed hope for a year ahead (the silver lining of January) is already beginning to wane. I'm pretty much crawling to the end of winter by this stage, and complaining about mud when I do. It's not a time I embrace; it's a time I loathe.

My mood and emotions can often plummet about now, and I get twitchy about wanting to leave Orkney because I'm so sick of the wind, rain, and dark. The only good thing about it is the excuse to hibernate. I often present as extrovert, and people naturally assume that I am. But my energy comes from solitude, quiet, calm, and being at one with the energy of the sea. After an often busy few weeks leading up to Christmas, I love the excuse to do very little in January and February. To go inwards and rest, napping on the couch in front of the fire on a harsh Sunday afternoon. Or read a book, drink tea from a favourite mug, and listen to the logs crackling as they burn. These are the good things, the things I love and appreciate.

And as I continued along with what I was now calling my best midlife crisis ever, wild swimming was also a good thing. Something in me was beginning to micro shift. Instead of assuming the horizontal position on a Sunday and whiling away several hours in slumber, I was opting for a sea swim with others, choosing icy waves over the warmth and comfort of the couch.

The local swim group often posts events and, while they can be completely random, there was a regular one posted at Tingwall harbour where the Orkney Polar Bears all began. On Sunday mornings, I now found myself getting up and heading down to the waves, instead of having a lie-in.

One particular Sunday, a swim event was posted at Yesnaby. This is a local beauty spot in Orkney, where waves crash against jagged cliffs positioned beautifully to catch the perfect sunset. In summer it is usually a popular campervan spot, and people can walk the edge of the cliffs and down the side to some coves. In winter it's a little more secluded and brooding, but still spectacular to view.

This was the first time I'd ever been to the cove, and it was a pretty windy ten-minute walk to access it. Once down there, we were more sheltered, and in order to enter the water you had to climb over stones and seaweed. For me, wild swimming was already becoming so much more than just swimming in the sea. There was the whole pilgrimage to the chosen spot, wanting to try new places, chatting as you walked down, accessing the water across sometimes difficult places, undignified falling over head-first into the water (it happens!), swimming in coves, adventuring in the most micro sense, but feeling like you've made a massive leap forwards in your own personal journey.

Wild swimming was breaking me out of a box I had no knowledge I'd been confined in. The first time I went to Yesnaby, the waters were wavy and we bounced around on them, all laughing our heads off. I can remember thinking this was without a doubt the best way to wake up on a Sunday morning. One time at Yesnaby, the waters were completely calm in the bay we swam, but as you looked out to the open waters you saw crashing waves just a few yards away. It really was the most remarkable sight, and I felt hugely privileged to be in the water to see something so indescribable in such a unique way.

Another time there, a seal swam backwards and forwards across the cove, just before the open water. We took it to be a sign of him marking his territory. We could swim so far but no further. We respected his space by keeping our distance, and as we left the water he stopped his border patrol and swam off. When there was no seal patrolling the territory, I was able to swim out a little further and explore the jagged cliffs and caves. Voices echoed off the cliffs and the wildness felt different and more thrilling. It quickly became my favourite spot. What the heck, they were all my favourite.

As much as I was finding so much joy in the water, I also remember lamenting the fact I had wasted so many years in Orkney and had never done this.

'It just wasn't your time,' a friend told me. This really struck a chord with me, and I had to forgive myself because it was so true. It wasn't my time for all those years. I had been single parenting for much of them, and now instead of a nest full of Lego, homework, exams, tears, and late nights listening for them to arrive home safely to their beds, I had a nest so empty it was hollow and giving off an agonising sound. My daughter (now aged 26) had left home several years before, but my son (now aged 20) had left only a few months ago, leaving a physical pain behind as I fretted and worried, but also as I marked the end of over 20 years of parenting at home. Empty nest syndrome was a thing, and I was feeling it as if it was grief. But this also freed up more space for me to do some of the things I had always promised myself I would do. Including things I clearly had no idea I wanted to do but was going to love.

'It just wasn't your time.' But now it was...

A friend told me she used to dedicate her swims

to someone when she journaled them. I thought this was the loveliest idea, and decided to do the same. Unfortunately for all its beauty, Yesnaby is also a local suicide spot where several cars have been driven over the top of its tall cliffs. Some of those people I have known.

Measures have been put in place to try and prevent this, but if a person is determined, they are determined. And it breaks my heart to think of the pain they must be in to do something so drastic. A few years ago, a young tourist guide accidentally fell off and died at Yesnaby whilst taking photographs – another tragedy. I decided to dedicate my swim there to all the people for whom Yesnaby is a source of pain. It felt very poignant, and in some small way a tiny mark of respect to the grieving friends and families.

Since starting, I'd always swum with a group and never alone. There is a hotly argued debate about lone swimming, and one that isn't going to be resolved in this book. Within reason, I do choose to swim alone from time to time, but always have certain safety measures in place. One being that I never go out of my depth when lone swimming, always making sure I can put my foot down and touch the bottom of the ocean. And I tend to avoid remote places, too, choosing somewhere I'm more visible.

I realise I'm a pretty risk-averse person, and I make no apology for that. I am who I am, and even though I've been somewhat ridiculed for opting out of swims, I would rather do that and regret it than opt in and live (or not!) to regret it. I'm not here to please anyone else, compete with anyone else, or garner any praise. I was doing this for my own journey – usually in company, but sometimes alone.

My first lone swim was mid-February, just some weeks after my initiation into the sea. I had woken crying, after dreaming about Mum. Following her diagnosis, we found ourselves in new territory.

Not much had actually changed; in fact, in a funny way, things had settled down a little. Mum was coming to terms with her diagnosis, but didn't need much help and could still function pretty well. I had provided a wipe clean memory board where Dad would write what day it was, what was for lunch and dinner, what appointments they had, and other things like that. It was proving successful for him at least, and we 'think' Mum was looking at it. She always claimed she did, but Dad light-heartedly claimed she didn't. Unbeknown to us, Mum had been worried silly that she was going to be 'locked up' when seen by the psychiatrist, and was hugely relieved when he let her go home.

But there had been other devastating news to contend with, and one of the hardest things for Mum to have to bear. As soon as she was diagnosed, she was told she was no longer allowed to drive. It was as immediate as that. If she had driven to hospital, she wasn't allowed to drive home. No more driving, forever.

Some people are allowed to drive with dementia. I don't know if it's the type of dementia they have, but

Mum's is associated with small strokes. The psychiatrist, who had been really lovely and kind, was also extremely determined that Mum was not to drive – and this was devastating for her. I printed off a form to surrender her licence to the DVLA, and Dad had the difficult task of asking her to give her licence to him so he could send it away. It was absolutely heartbreaking, and she sobbed and sobbed.

The loss of independence was tough to bear, and I vividly remember Mum standing in the kitchen saying, 'I've been driving for 60 years, I know how to drive!' It was true; she had and she did. But what if she drove and had a lapse, not knowing where she was? Or made a momentary error with lasting effects involving her or someone else? It didn't bear thinking about, and in the months it took for Mum to come to terms with not driving, I was absolutely worried sick.

In the early days, she claimed she would drive if she had to in an emergency, and I was genuinely ill with worry that she would. Through many situations, I oscillated between not wanting to remove her rights and dignity and not wanting her to bring harm to herself or someone else. She struggled to understand that although she could drive, she was no longer legal to drive as she had relinquished her licence. I tried to explain that it would be the same as a drunk driver getting behind the wheel, or someone without insurance. None of it worked. I just had to hope and pray that there would never be such an emergency, and thankfully there never has been.

All this driving angst and loss was playing heavy on my heart at the time, and it had spilled over into my dreams. I can remember waking, having had the most vivid dream about Mum. She was young and without dementia. The mum of my childhood. But in the dream, she was out of my reach; as I put my hand out, I couldn't touch her or hold her hand. I could only look at her from a distance. It was heartbreaking, and the tears in my dream spilled over into my waking.

As I opened my eyes, it was an unusually spring-like February morning. The sun was streaming in the window and I had a rare day off from work. I decided I needed the ocean to wash away my sadness, so I jumped in the car to the local beach. As the crow flies, I would be there in minutes, yet in the car it's a mile-and-a-half. Soon I was parked up. It was my first lone swim, and I didn't plan to stay long.

I headed across the stones and splashed into the waves. Nothing sharpens your focus like an icy blast from a wave, and as you catch your breath and put your shoulders under, you are totally in the moment and think of nothing else but where you are. There's no place for distraction, no space for the rest of life. It's just you, the waves, the cold, the salt, and the moment. That moment might only be ten or 15 minutes, but it's yours, it's exhilarating, and the effects can last for hours. The tears I thought I might drown in were washed away by a different kind of saltwater. I returned home reset. I had this. I could do hard things.

By the time I reached my 21st swim, I was out of my wetsuit and swimming skins. People had given me tips for coming out of a wetsuit. For example, in order to acclimatise some swimmers unzip their wetsuit and take the top half down for the last minute or so of their swim. I tried this, and it was still intolerable. It was just too cold, and I wasn't ready. As a compromise, I ordered some neoprene leggings and a zip-up rash vest which had a neoprene body and thin nylon arms. It was one millimetre thinner than what I'd been using, and I was amazed at the difference 1mm less makes but it was a start.

The downside of a wetsuit is it can be a hassle taking off once out the water. I seemed to spend half my time pulling and tugging at the legs to get my feet out, and none of this is easy when the air temp could freeze the balls of an Eskimo. You also had to rinse it and dry it, so there was a fair amount of maintenance admin to complete as well. And for a lazy oik like me, this all added to the hassle. I was desperate to streamline the process, but not so desperate to swim skins. But once I went skins, I never went back to a wetsuit of any kind.

In the end, it happened quite by accident. I'd forgotten to rinse and dry my things from my day's swim and was heading out to a swim the following day. I quickly realised that by the time I'd finished faffing about on the side of the water putting on a wet wetsuit, I might as well just discard it and swim skins. I don't mind admitting I was terrified to begin with, but I watched other people and decided if they could do it so could I.

We were swimming at Tingwall that morning. A small pier where a boat carrying passengers to and from Rousay is used daily, and where several fishing boats land their catch. It has a slip, access is easy, and it can either be very bouncy or sheltered depending on the wind direction. So, wearing only a swimsuit, neoprene gloves and shoes, I bit the bullet, waded in, and swam into the six-degree water.

When you enter the cold water, you immediately put your body under slight stress, forcing it into the fight or flight mode. Your blood rushes to your organs to protect them, and the first blast takes your breath away. Then you start to swim, and within a minute or so you have adapted to the water. And although cold, something magical is happening. Endorphins are being released (endolphins, as we fondly call them) and you get the cold water high that all ice swimmers are chasing. Amazingly, you are able to adjust and cope with the cold. We truly are remarkable creatures.

I remember walking down the slip and being so nervous that it almost felt like starting this craziness all over again from day one. I don't know if it was adrenaline or a cosmic shift in my brain, but unlike other times when I'd tried it, this time it really was fine. I let the magic happen, and came out feeling high as a kite, which lasted the entire day. I had always found myself a little too buoyant in the wetsuit, but in a swimsuit it was much more like normal. And it was good to feel the water, and the salt, properly against my skin. Just like that, another skins swimmer was born.

For the first time in my life, I finished February in a completely different place than usual. Wild swimming had rescued me from the claws of winter and turned my loathing into loving. And it was growing in popularity, both in Orkney and nationally. I knew I was in vogue when I saw wild swimming featured on *Songs of Praise* a few weeks before, and due to my evangelising on social media, people were regularly stopping me and asking me about it, wanting to know if they could join me to give it a try.

I was always happy to help someone along into the sea if they wanted to give it a try, as people had been so supportive with me, and there was a flurry of new sea swimmers popping up everywhere. A couple of folk implied that people were only doing it because it was popular and to be seen, but for me that was a ridiculous thing to say. People enjoying fresh air and activity was a good thing, surely? And I was certainly doing that.

They could make walking popular and I would still not want to walk from the house to the car, because for me there was no buzz. I really couldn't see how getting into such cold water because it was 'in' would last. Those that were possibly doing it for that reason would eventually tail off. And as the months went by, they did. But anyone who thought I was doing it for the hype, clearly didn't know me. I was doing it because I now had a four times-a-week habit, and rising. I guess one person's wild swimming addiction is another person's Candy Crush, but I was well and truly hooked, and loving every second of it.

March

Well, this is exciting! It's International Mermaid Day, and what could be more suited to me? In honour of such a special day, I'm going to wear a crown, sing underwater, accessorise with shells (note to self, find bigger shell bra,) and sit staring dreamily out to sea while my real life actual fisherman husband looks on mesmerised by my charm and beauty. (Might lure him to his death by my singing if he continues to put the toilet roll on the wrong way round!)

(Instagram @seasaltandsarah)

The battle between winter and spring had begun, and there would be many skirmishes before spring finally arrived to restore us. My beloved snowdrops were everywhere as March began, and would eventually give way to an explosion of yellow as the daffodil soldiers arrived for the final winter/spring smackdown. There was a smattering of 'lambing snow' – a wet snow that is the final whimper as winter dies, and many Orcadians will not allow spring to be mentioned until lambing snow is by. I was once keen and excited at the sight of a spring morning and voiced it to a friend, only to be told it wasn't spring yet because we'd not had the lambing snow.

The water tells a rather different story. And rather than beginning to warm up, it is often one or two degrees colder in February and March. The coldest for me was 4.5 degrees, but someone else measured 3.8 degrees where they swam. Our remarkably resilient bodies keep doing their thing and, as a group, one of the first things we all do is estimate the temperature before someone pulls out a thermometer from the front of their costume (fondly known as a boobometer by some) and gives the final reading. It's amazing how accurate we can be, and often our estimate is only out by one or half a degree. I'll know we have gone below seven degrees by the amount it takes my breath away and the discomfort I feel when I first swim. By the time it gets to five degrees or below, the discomfort has become pain for sixty seconds.

Mothering Sunday almost always falls in March, and this year my daughter shared a photo on social media of a much younger me holding her. I remember the photo being taken, where we were, and the friend taking it. Katie was less than five months old, and my journey into mothering was just beginning. Of course, in those days it was a photo with a camera, not a phone, and you waited weeks whilst you used the film up, then sent it away. Your photos were then developed and returned with stickers on them to tell you where it all went wrong.

As I look back at the photo, I can't believe how young my hands look. I'm almost horrified at the difference between then and now; the lifetime of mother jobs that my hands have seen in between. Driving to singing lessons, dance school, ballet, work, Boys' Brigade; Santa; grazed knees; fancy dress costumes; homework; school plays; sledging; feeding the ducks, don't touch; meningitis; appendix out; taking temperatures; Calpol; swimming; this club, that club; no you can't, yes you can; it's chicken for tea; stop fighting; I love you; I will always love you; three more mouthfuls; night, night, sleep tight, don't let the bedbugs bite; pushchairs; car seats; washing, washing, washing; parents' evenings; two more sleeps; orthodontist; church; Sunday school; parties; chasing away nightmares; bath time; washing, washing, washing; 'what's for tea?' (it's still chicken); library; Beavers; Cubs; Brownies; college applications; driving lessons; listening for their arrival home; theory tests; struggles; successes; and love, love, love.

I've changed nappies, wiped noses, dried tears, read stories, cured hiccups, cooked meals, cleaned up sick, driven to hospital, wrapped presents, held hands, listened, talked, laughed, and cried an ocean of tears at the enormity of it all. I know my children better than I know anyone else. I've counted their eyelashes, fingers, and toes, as they lay cradled in my arms, and know their faces better than I know my own.

I cannot ever imagine looking at their beautiful faces and not recognising them. They are my life; I adore them.

How can it be possible that a parent can come to a stage that they don't recognise their child? This hasn't happened between Mum and I, and hopefully might never. But I know it happens time and time again to others, and I'm already anxiously waiting for the axe to fall.

By March, I was taking every opportunity to swim, and as there was a chink more light at the end of the day, the chance of swimming after work was becoming more real.

A swim was planned with the group, and I was looking forward to it. I went along to the chosen space and checked the event on Facebook to see who else was coming. One by one, others had cancelled, and I realised to my frustration that the swim was not going ahead. It happens – people get ill, have appointments, and are busy – but I sat in the car and cried. I actually cried because a swim in the sea had been cancelled.

I drove away upset and agitated, and I knew my response was so ridiculously out of proportion to the disappointment and incredibly first world problematic. Driving home, I was scanning the water all the way and knew there was a secluded spot where I could sneak into the sea for a quick dip. So, I took a detour and headed to the beach, telling myself it was 'just for a look'.

By the time I arrived at the beach, the light was fading, and I hastily changed into my costume in the car, feeling guilty. *No-one knows I'm here; I'm becoming secretive; I shouldn't be doing this alone; people would disapprove.* But I had to get in.

43

I made my way down to the sea, feeling a mixture of exhilaration and guilt. I was in the water in seconds and let out a gasp as the cold hit me. The relief was enormous, and I was instantly calmed. I felt better, I was settled, I was restored. I stayed long enough to satisfy my soul, but left before it was too dark to see my way back up the beach to the car. A short swim, but one packed with learning, as I knew I'd taken a risk – one my husband wouldn't approve of.

Respecting the sea is the most vital and important part of this hobby, and whilst I never went out of my depth, I knew by my feelings that this wasn't a calculated thing but a response to a need to do this to calm my agitation. I dedicated this swim to myself. I was full of life, full of light, happy and free. I also went home and ordered myself a tow float – a high visible inflatable that is attached to your waist via a belt, and floats along behind you. It was the least I could do to minimise the danger from my fast-growing addictive behaviour.

Mum and Dad had booked a holiday for March, months before Mum had a diagnosis and before we really knew anything was going wrong. It was a regular place in Lanzarote, and the same hotel they knew and loved. This time, they had invited me and my husband Roy (often nicknamed Orkney Beef on my social media posts and blog) to go along for the second week. I hadn't been abroad in years and neither had Roy.

We had a wonderful time and swam daily in the sea. Surprisingly, the cold took your breath away just as always on entry, but the adjustment took a second rather than 60, and the water was so much warmer. I was delirious to stay in for sometimes an hour, snorkelling with my husband by my side for once.

Mum was happy on holiday, but we had to put slight measures in place to ensure she was safe and ok. At dinner time she would go to the buffet and choose her food then forget where her table was to return to. She didn't feel she needed hand-holding, but it worried Dad, so we took it in turns to keep a watchful eye out for her, and someone always stayed at the table so she could spot us easily.

Small things can often signify a significant shift, and one morning I asked Mum if she wanted to sit by the pool or walk down to the beach. 'I don't know. I'm just waiting to be told what to do. Tell me what to do,' she replied.

My heart sank that my strong, assertive, and decisive Mothership was now unable to make a decision about how to spend her holiday time. But with the sadness, there was a relief that she was so amenable and calm.

Mum and Dad have always held hands wherever they go, and holiday time was no different. I loved seeing the tenderness my dad showed Mum. He was totally devoted to her enjoying her holiday in the sun; it brings a lump to my throat as I think back.

Returning to Orkney meant a drop in the water temperature from 21 degrees to 6 degrees, and I felt extremely nervous once again. Not wanting to give up my hobby, I knew I just had to get back in and get on with it. So the day after I arrived home, I was back in the water and more than surprised that I preferred the cold. So strange; it must be the endolphins! This thing I'd found was exhilarating and wonderful, and the sea was always there for me, waiting for me to join it whenever I could, and healing me each time. Healing comes in waves, both figuratively and literally.

April

Nothing recalibrates me like a dip in the sea, so I always carry my swim gear in the car just in case the conditions are right. Tonight, my beloved Skaill was flat calm and I had a beautiful solitary swim en route home from work. A curious gull skimmed right across the water close to me, a fisherman waved. Be still my soul.

(Diary entry)

I f I was on commission for encouraging people to give this new activity a try, I'd be wealthy enough to give up work and be acting like a dog with two tails. Not because money is everything, but because I'd finally have the time to finish my crochet blanket. I started it several centuries ago, and the next available opportunity is when I retire, which apparently is something people used to do in the old days before we had to keep working until we reached 100 or died, whichever comes first. Ignore me, I'm on a rant!

I wasn't asking people to join me. I was just absolutely high on my new and brilliant hobby and couldn't stop evangelising about it, so they started asking me. I started to write a blog where I uploaded new pictures every week. I also shared these on social media and chatted with other swimmers about our swims. Non-wild swimmers were naturally curious and asked me about it, with more and more people seeming to want to give it a try. The majority of people who decide they want to give it a go, end up sticking with it. As I've discovered, it's rarely something people do once.

And there are so many benefits to swimming in the sea: it relieves stress; boosts the immune system and circulation; and I was beginning to notice my skin was now so soft. The skin absorbs nutrients from the sea such as magnesium, calcium, potassium, and sodium. An added bonus was that the arthritis pain I'd been getting in my fingers and elbows was almost completely gone. This might not be the case for everyone – we are all different – but for me, the cold water and movement was a huge benefit in pain relief without needing medication. Research seems to be mainly anecdotal but so many people say the same thing, yet despite the well documented benefits, there are certain sea delights that repeatedly put people off.

Aside from the cold, the two things most commonly referred to as less than desirable are seaweed and the unknown entity of what lies beneath – unknown sea monsters, sharks, seals, and Ursula the sea witch. People just don't like the thought of unidentifiable things touching them in the water. It seems they have vivid imaginations, and so do I when caught off guard. I once screamed thinking I'd seen a shark's fin, and it turned out to be someone's foot.

Another time I was snorkelling in my lunch break (as you do) and I felt something touch me. Exploring underwater can be exciting but also a little bit creepy, so I bobbed up quickly and began acting out the scene from Jaws, only to discover my own tow float had touched me. These hi-vis safety devices are made to store your valuables inside, like a phone and car keys, and are designed to make you more visible to jet skis or fishing boats, etc. They can also double up as pretend sharks when imagination is running a little too high.

I never once gave sharks a thought until people kept asking about sharks, which was a little disconcerting. Equally, I wasn't bothered by seaweed touching me, then I realised I hadn't felt it touch me initially because I'd always been in a wetsuit. The first time I swam skins, I let out a screech when I swam over the top of the floating garden. I actually shouted out loud, 'Ursula the sea witch just grabbed my ankle', as the spaghetti seaweed brushed past my leg. Maybe I was being a tad dramatic.

Once a friend I'd made over social media suggested we meet up for a swim, so we went to Inganess and swam around the wreck. Swimming round the *Juniata* is a rite of passage for Orkney sea swimmers, and one that made me slightly nervous the first time. It looks quite foreboding as it sits staring out at you in silence on each visit.

My intention was to swim up to it and back, but I was encouraged to go around with some more experienced swimmers, and it took me 23 minutes from start to finish, swimming at high tide. As I swam with this friend, I knew she wasn't a fan of seaweed, so as we approached the boat, I advised her to go wide as there was a big patch that I pointed to. She not only went wide; she was off like a rocket and I couldn't keep up. My pointing out the seaweed patch was enough to make her go as fast as I can mainline a packet of biscuits when stress-eating. And, readers, that's fast! I found it really endearing when I finally caught her up.

Another friend, Ally, who wanted to join me and started sea swimming in April, absolutely hated the idea of seaweed touching her. We had walked to a new swim spot together, and it had been a bit of a trek to reach. It was a beautiful secluded bay near the fishermen's huts – stone-built huts dating back over 100 years, built into the landscape for fishermen to take shelter or to store things. They are long since disused, but now forever etched into the landscape's history.

I was in the water before her, and realised there was no way in other than wading through a massive amount of seaweed. I turned around and broke the news to her. 'You're just going to have to get over it, Ally, there's nowhere clear to go in. But once you're past it, it's fine!' I shouted from the sea.

'It's just a vegetable,' shouted our other swimming companion, as she bounced in the waves.

'I'm going to quote you in my book!' I shouted back as we all laughed.

Ally got over her fear of the sea vegetable, and grew to love it with a passion. So much so, she now spends much of her time studying it and photographing it, and even making artwork from it. Who knows what can come of us if we face our fears?

Even though seaweed never bothered me, I've had my moments of speeding up when a seal comes too close. I was once swimming with a large group when someone spotted a seal pretty near us. I was furthest out, so speed-swam in. The group were laughing at my playful distress, and one of them reassured the rest of the group that they were safe.

'Don't worry, they pick off the weak ones at the back,' she joked across to me, and there was a collective laugh and a faster swim from me.

The social element to wild swimming is one of the most enjoyable parts for me. I've swum with one or two, and swum in big groups. If I want to swim hard, I go to the pool and plough up and down doing lengths. If I want to chat, enjoy the great outdoors and the sensory aspect of cold water, I swim wild and meet up with like-minded people.

Connection with people works in a different way from meeting up for a drink in a pub or going for a walk together. There's often bite-sized conversations, and no topic is left undiscussed. There's a rhythm to conversation that takes on a familiar regularity. The temperature is always number one, which moves on to the sea state, wildlife, decisions about which direction to swim to, and general chit chat. In the sea, all manner of things are discussed: relationships, career paths, child-rearing, pets, house redecorating, swimsuits, weight, TV shows, housework, needlecraft, washing, social media, books, TV shows, aging bodies, and ageing parents. There is always laughter.

I was in my happy place and spamming everyone to death with pictures and talk of wild swimming. I had become a complete wild swimming bore. The car was permanently smelling of damp swimming stuff, and covered in a layer of sand. I was absolutely winning at life, looking well, and feeling amazing. I was now choosing wild swimming over pool swimming as often as I could, and loving every experience. The first time I had a before-work swim was absolutely incredible for me. I met a friend at a local swim spot at 7.30am and swam for about 25 minutes, before dressing quickly and heading into work. It was so empowering and something we did a lot of for a few months, and something I truly loved. In the pool, I don't need to speak to anyone; in the sea, I love the companionship. The cold water is such a tiny part of the experience, and is simply one of many elements that makes sea swimming so wonderful. Oh, why did I wait so long?

This whole thing started because I'd been wanting to do the 49 things while I was still 49, and I'd become side-tracked very quickly. I was still working through a list of things and looking for ideas of experiences to try, but not one of them captured me the way sea swimming did.

I'd been following an account of Orkney rowers and they had offered an opportunity for new people to go along, so one Sunday morning I gave it a go and absolutely sucked at it. I 'caught the crab' twice. This is where the oar hits the water at a wrong angle and gets 'caught', nearly launching me over the side of the boat. I was less than dignified and went flying off the seat, nearly landing in the lap of the person behind me. It was hilariously funny, and everyone was very patient and encouraging, but I never went back to it.

I also saw a calf being born. A friend and colleague was married to a farmer, and lived near to me. I had spoken about wanting to see a calf being born, and one Saturday evening I was making tea and received the following message: 'Coo calving' (Coo being Orcadian for cow). So, tea was abandoned, and I raced over to hers in time for the delivery. I was amazed at how quiet and peaceful the cow was when giving birth, and commented on it. I was told it was self-preservation, as a cow is so vulnerable when calving that if they were making a noise they would expose themselves to any predator.

My friend said when she was in labour herself, her farmer husband turned to her and said, 'Honestly, Gillian, you couldnae have a coo walking about the field making that racket!' Probably not the wisest thing to say to a woman in labour, but very funny nevertheless.

There were other joyful by-products of sea swimming, too. I absolutely love mooching about the beach picking up pieces of china and sea glass, as well as shells. The china is my favourite, though. To find a piece of patterned china means it had a story, it was once something, it had journeyed across the ocean to be washed up on the beach – from where? I loved imagining the stories behind each piece, and frequently filled my pockets with the china to take it to its final resting place in a glass vase on my bathroom windowsill.

Many Orkney people take delight in Groatie Buckie hunting. Groatie Buckies are little cowrie shells that are hard to find and considered to be lucky. One friend took great delight in searching for these shells. She told me it helped her cope with the loss of her lifelong partner, the mindfulness of it a sheer relaxation. I don't mind the occasional mooch, but have no connection to them and have been known to chuck them away before now – something which will make Orkney readers gasp and one or two never forgive me. But when a friend referred to my sea swimming journey as 'You've found your Groatie Buckies', I knew exactly what she meant.

I was finding great joy in being at one with nature, and now daily light was increasing, I had an overwhelming sense of wellbeing. Roy wasn't yet ready to join me in the sea. Being a fisherman for many years, he'd had his share of being in the water – sometimes unplanned. But occasionally he came along and took the dog, throwing the ball into the sea for her to fetch time and time again.

Once he threw it too far and the dog was unable to retrieve it, so I had to swim out and rescue it. 'This is practically Baywatch,' I said, turning to my friend. And oh, how we laughed.

Despite the ever-increasing infectious joy I found from this hobby-come-obsession, there was still a heaviness in the pit of my stomach. It was like carrying a stone around with me all the time. A stone in itself might not necessarily be heavy, but when you have it with you constantly and you're never allowed to set it down, it can become that way.

Usually the stone felt enough to manage. I knew it was there; I could see it, acknowledge it, and recognise the stone as my living grief for the changes I was seeing in my mum. But it was becoming heavier. Some days, I felt barely able to lift it, and I could certainly never leave it behind. Wherever I went, the stone came, too, and I would frequently cry on my way over to Mum and Dad's house to visit, or on my way home as the stone reminded me of its presence. The stone made me feel sad, angry, grief-stricken, and anxious.

Despite crying on the five-mile journey to my parents, I always forced myself together so that I could be upbeat and of some use when I got there. As I turned the corner to pull into their drive, I knew it was time to take deep breaths, dry my tears, and smile. We would go for a walk if the weather was decent, but one time on a walk with Mum, I couldn't hold back the tears any longer. As we walked along the track road to the whalebone – Dad's favourite spot in the whole of Orkney, and minutes away from my parents' house – the choking sobs burst out.

Mum turned to me saying, 'Don't upset yourself, darling. I'm still the same person, I think I've just worn my brain out.' She looked at me, wiped my tears, and hugged me.

As we embraced, I locked the memory away in my mind forever, and we continued on our walk, me dragging the stone behind.

May

Lunchtime dilemma. Do I stay in front of the computer and go home in the shape of the chair, or join like-minded sea swimming lovers and go home in the shape of the sea? No brainer.

(Instagram @seasaltandsarah)

When I first married my husband, he was a fisherman. And I loved it when he was home from a day's work, because I could still smell the sea in his hair. Now through my new connection with cold water, I could smell it on my own hair.

Smell is such a powerful sense, evoking so many memories. If I smell face powder, I am reminded of hugging Mum as a child, and I am transported back to her bedroom, playing with the compact on her dressing table. The smell of Milton disinfectant instantly takes me back to 2am feeds over 26 years ago, when all we had to sterilise dummies and bottles was a big plastic container filled with water and Milton. Boiled cabbage – my first tiny flat when the man across the hall seemed to live off it; fried onions – fairgrounds. And the smell of the sea

57

takes me back to childhood holidays and a longing for waves.

As I look back over my year of wild swimming, May was when I was at my peak. I still considered myself a newbie, and I was yet to swim through a winter, even though I started in January. However, I had enough swims under my belt to really make this a wonderful and worthwhile hobby. It was accessible, free, and something I could easily slot into my life, be it before or after work, or even in a lunch break.

The days were full of light and warmth, and I now had a permanent suntan, which I'm sure came from the reflection of the sun on the salty water. It was something people commented on all the time. Water temperatures were warming slightly, and I seemed to be swimming constantly. I even swam three times one Friday, as people posted 'anyone up for a swim' events and I just couldn't resist saying no. We would swim in groups, or sometimes one or two of us. Sometimes we swam hard, other times we mucked around, diving into the weekend full of joy, people playfully splashing in waves, doing handstands. It was all fun and games until someone got an ice cream headache.

Admittedly, I was tired by the end of the day, but I was learning to grab at opportunities and had a new-found love for being outdoors and connecting with nature. I was pushing myself to new limits all the time. Going for a daily swim outdoors was now as natural to me as walking the dog.

I felt a slight sense of betrayal towards the swimming pool that had been my friend for so long, having gone there four or five times a week before work for nearly the last two years. But my desire to be outside among beautiful nature and surroundings was now winning every time.

I'd grown quite used to gulls skimming the water in front of me as I swam, and oyster catchers are a common sight in Orkney frequenting the beaches and taking flight in huge groups as we approached the water's edge. I'd swum near beautiful arctic terns, curlews, fulmars, shags, eider ducks and swans.

On a rare occasion when Roy swam with me, he reminded me that we are in their environment not them in ours. This conversation took place as we were out swimming locally, and swans headed towards us. He told me to change direction so that we were no threat to them, which we did, and the swans swam away again. It was a timely reminder to continually respect the ocean and nature that we were enjoying.

Where I could, I would pick up rubbish from the beach on my way back to the car. There's an alarming increase in plastic waste washed up on the shores, and it seems a never-ending task to try and keep up with it. Orkney has an annual 'Bag the Bruck' event, when volunteers go out and clean up the beaches of everything washed in by the tide.

I actually find it quite soothing walking along with a bag and collecting the rubbish, but it also saddens my heart to see it. The weirdest thing I found was an onion sitting on the shoreline, but over the years I've seen all sorts of things washed in by the tide, covered in barnacles, sometimes too heavy to lift, like a tractor tyre, before the tide reclaimed it for her own again some weeks later.

The ocean was now my second home and I was unintentionally creating my own swimming 'bucket list' of things and places to try. A moonlit swim, a new spot or point-to-point, round the wreck in the dark. I was so keen to experience everything, and sometimes that came with a cost… like setting my alarm at stupid o'clock.

The first of May is an important day in the Celtic calendar, as it signifies the return of summer. Washing your face in the morning dew is an ancient tradition which is supposed to aid health, happiness, and youthful looks. It would take a powerful dew to keep me looking youthful, but it's still something I take part in for the fun of it. I enjoy connecting with my ancestors' rituals to keep them alive.

In ancient days, Beltane festivals took place on May 1st as people said goodbye to the darkness, welcomed the new light, and signalled animals going out to pasture. This involved much celebration, fires, and even human sacrifices. Human sacrifice was NOT something I wanted to connect with, but as a nod to the joy of summer returning, I was happy to take part in a sunrise swim on this first day of May. I would later discover it was something commonplace in the outdoor swimming community, through the enormity of photos that appeared on social media.

I rose at 4.20am to be at the beach for sunrise, which was just after 5am. It was about 25 minutes' drive away, and four of us met up to swim there while a bigger group met at a location further way on the island. It was dark as I got into my car, but light was beginning to show itself by the time we were ready to swim.

We swam at Evie – a beach I'd swum at several times. But being here while the world slept was absolutely magical. It was misty, calm, and totally serene. The tranquillity was breathtaking, and while we swam we chatted in low voices not wanting to break the magic.

'Seal!' someone said in an excited whisper. As usual, a curious sea dog had stuck his head up near to us to investigate, and we all trod water silently, looking at him looking at us as he bobbed up, watched, and disappeared again, only to bob up again elsewhere. Trying to catch one on camera in the sea is a nightmare. It's like a game of whack-a-mole, as heads bob up and down in curiosity. Despite many attempts, I've never managed to photograph a seal whilst in the water.

We swam back to the shore, and as we approached I could see the tide had come in fast. I'd set my phone up on a tripod to time lapse our swim, as I commonly do. The sea was now lapping the bottom of my phone, and I went flying out of the sea at great speed and managed to rescue it just in the nick of time. I laughed and said it was old and I was due a new one anyway.

We dried and dressed quickly, and on my drive home I had that familiar high as my body began to warm up again from the cold. For some reason, this remains one of my most memorable swims. It was atmospheric and magical, smooth, tranquil, quiet, and peaceful.

As I drove away from the swim, I reflected on what I'd just done, shaking my head at the thought of me getting up before 4.30am just to swim. 'You've lost your mind!' I said out loud. But the sea didn't reply, it simply waved. When I arrived home, I was exuberant, and my heart was full. I had never felt so alive.

To add to the insanity, we all decided we wanted to be in the water for sunset, too, on 1st May. So back we went to a good sunset location for a double dip day. Life was a constant round of getting cold in the water and warming up again, but I was having the best time.

Orkney has a saying, 'Ne'er cast a cloot 'til May be oot' which loosely translates to 'don't go anywhere without a coat until May is over with'. And then, still don't go anywhere without a coat in Orkney... ever. Because the weather cannot be relied upon, and you're highly likely to be caught out one of these days. (Note, I may have embellished the true sentiment of the saying a tiny bit).

I've ignored this wisdom many times, mainly because I can be a bit of a scatterbrain and just forget to take a coat. I once went for a walk on a beautiful May morning. On seeing how sunny it was outside, I decided on a lightweight hi-vis top, and my waterproof breeks were cast aside with joyful abandon. Off I set, striding out, and listening to my various podcast choices.

I bumped into neighbours and passed the time of day before continuing on my journey. The sun was shining, the dog was happy, and I was full of the potential of spring just around the corner. I arrived at my destination, which was about two miles from home. The dog ran along the beach and I surveyed the damage from the storms earlier in the week. Tons of seaweed mountains had been washed in with giant waves, and litter was strewn everywhere, a ton of plastic vomited up by the sea.

I started to make my way back up the road and the heavens opened, soaking me with icy cold rain within seconds. I was in the middle of nowhere, frozen to the very core, water dripping off my hair, shivering, miserable, and on the verge of tears. Admitting defeat, I went to call Roy and ask him to come and pick me up, but to my horror there was no signal. Not even the tiniest glimmer of half a bar. Absolute zilch.

All I had to take my mind off things was a podcast I was listening to: The benefits of walking. You couldn't make this stuff up, could you? After the hailstorm eased off, I trudged back up the road, legs raw with cold, teeth chattering, hair dripping wet, and made straight for a hot shower. Several hours later, I still hadn't warmed up.

As much as I love being cold in the water, I hate being cold out of it. I'm sure there are regular silent battles in every household, and ours is the same. I leave lights on,

Roy turns them off; Roy puts the toilet roll on the wrong way round, I turn it the correct way (see also loading dishwasher – it's enough to break a couple); and I loathe going to bed in a cold bedroom, while Roy hates it too warm.

I'm from the era where you woke up to ice on the inside of the window, so now a bit of warmth is a deal-breaker for me. 'Sarah, you swim in freezing cold sea almost every day and then complain about being cold and flick on the heating constantly,' he once said to me.

'Yeah well, I'm a girl and I can do whatever I want,' I replied whilst casually flicking on the heating.

Heck, as I watched the sea disappear from view under a blanket of fog one day in May, I even contemplated getting the mulled wine going.

The weather could be changeable, and I found myself asking how I could be swimming in sunglasses at the beginning of the week and in a hailstorm by the end of it. Hailstones are painful when you're dashing out of the water and racing to the car, even on numb skin, but nothing was more painful than my one and only swim where I left the water in a worse mood than when I went in.

It was May 28th, according to my diary, and I was swimming before work at the local place we call The Choin. As the tide recedes, we find a giant lagoon, and it's great for swimming safely, while surfers prefer to be the other side of the reef. I had stopped wearing neoprene gloves, having forgotten them once several weeks before, and I realised I could manage without them now the water was three or four degrees higher.

The swim was fine and we were enjoying ourselves, but from nowhere the wind picked up, making the waters choppy and the wind chill biting. It was time to get out, and during the process my hands became very cold. I've never known cold like it, and they wouldn't and couldn't function. I managed to get the car door open and drove the short distance home in my towelling robe and change robe, then headed into the shower, making pathetic whimpering sounds as I tried to restore feeling back into my fingers. I cried with pain in the shower, and whilst I continued to swim without gloves in the summer months, I returned to them in the autumn as the waters cooled down again. Although I've known cold hands since, I've never experienced anything like that painful and memorable day in May. Life is a rollercoaster, it seems, even with wild swimming.

All in all, from a swimming perspective, May was a glorious month. Bluebells were out in full force, I was trying new things and enjoying lighter evenings, I was feeling and sleeping much better, and a transformation was taking place. So much so that for Mental Health Awareness Week I decided to post the following caption on my social media, along with a photo.

taps mic nervously I'm currently almost daily swimming in the sea, an activity I intended to do as a one-off in January this year, but was instantly hooked. I feel so much better and look so much better. (I only know this because people tell me every single day how well I look.) My 49-year-old self has a healthy glow and, despite a multitude of grey hairs appearing, I feel pretty good about myself. But as it's #mentalhealthawarenessweek, I wanted to tell you the story behind the 49-year-old me. From the age of 24-39 I was on and off antidepressants on a regular basis. I was signed off work with depression, sometimes for several months. I cried daily. I didn't wear makeup for years. I lacked motivation. I struggled my way through life as a single mum. I was desperately lonely. I was hard on myself. I had little self-worth, and thought I would be stuck like this forever. I would put on a brave face and have always had the ability to make people laugh, but the reality was it was all a major struggle. If I could talk to my younger self, I would be kind to her. I'd tell her what an amazingly strong woman she would turn out to be. I'd tell her she can do the things she never thought she would. That she will still be a sensitive soul, but that's ok. I'd tell her that eventually she will stop crying. Eventually she will emerge and be able to function and contribute and be a much better self. I would tell my younger self that she was doing her best, and it was fabulous. Sometimes I need to tell my older self that, too! People often describe me as bubbly and outgoing, but in reality I need my solitude and calm and quiet to survive. Solitude is a lifeline to me and I'm self-aware enough to know this and to know what self-care I need if things get stressful. What I'm ultimately trying to say is this: Your now picture is not your forever picture. You may be going through the worst of times, but it won't be like this forever. My younger self could never have imagined how my older self would turn out to be. Now, please do me a favour and tag someone you think needs to read this, cos I'm genuinely having butterflies & feel a bit sick about uploading. But it might just help someone.

Your now picture is not your forever picture.

Read that again.

Your now picture is not your forever picture.

I need to read that again.

My now picture is not my forever picture.

I say this phrase to so many people when they are going through hard times, and I often have to say it back to myself when the road gets bumpy. I know from bitter experience that what can seem like an eternal dark tunnel will eventually open out into the light, if you can just keep going.

★

Mum was ticking over, but cracks were beginning to appear as her condition worsened at a speed we weren't expecting.

There can be a lot of commonality among people with dementia, but each case is individual, too. Mum's official diagnosis was Multi-Infarct Vascular Dementia, and from our understanding this meant she would go down in steps rather than a gradual decline. But even so, we didn't really know what that would look like in the long term.

She would cry frequently, and this emotion is part of the condition. Naturally, we want to ask, 'Why are you crying?' But it's so difficult for her to explain, as the words disappear and thoughts vanish along with them.

We naturally want to fix an upset person, but dementia is unfixable. It can sometimes be slowed down by medication, depending on the type of dementia a person has, but the reality is dementia is a one-way street that feels long, empty, and lonely, both for the sufferer and the loved ones. Seeing my mum cry, while my dad bravely stood by her side helping all he could, was absolutely heartbreaking.

My sister living across the world was heartbroken, too, and managed a visit twice a year, but travelling here was expensive and time-consuming, often involving three flights. She would FaceTime our parents regularly, and then the iPad would malfunction, Mum would try to retrieve it, lock herself out, I would go over and sort it, repeat, repeat, repeat.

I watched Mum struggling to find words, clawing at them, trying to bring them to the surface, only to have them disappear like smoke. She was slowly beginning to lose track of things in the kitchen. 'I can't find where the cake forks go,' she told me once as she stood with them in her hand. We laughed that, despite everything, at least we were still posh enough to use cake forks.

I was doing things intentionally to try to make memories for myself and create happy feelings for Mum. Even if she didn't recall having done something or been somewhere, at least she would be enjoying the moment, and I was benefitting from time spent with her, while Dad could get a little break. As much as he needed a break sometimes, he pined for her in equal measure. I once took Mum for a walk around the shops and a coffee, leaving Dad to rest for a few hours. When we arrived home, he was at the door before we were out of the car, longing for his wife to be home. Their love for each other was and always has been a privilege to see.

A really special memory was made in May. It started circa 1974 when I was a very little girl and completely in love with ballet. I would watch it any opportunity and dance to a vinyl record of ballet favourites that Dad had. So great was my passion that for my birthday Mum took me to the ballet at a theatre in Birmingham. I absolutely loved it, and still treasure that time some 45 years later.

As the Royal Opera House now live streams ballets and operas to cinemas around the world, I took the opportunity to take Mum to the ballet in return. It was at our local cinema in Orkney, and all the way there Mum kept asking where we were going – another signal that her short-term memory was failing. She herself would often say she felt bewildered. But when we arrived it was all worth it, as we sat side-by-side and watched an exquisite performance of *Romeo and Juliet*. As we waited for the performance to start, patriotic music was being played and Mum sang *Land of Hope and Glory* with great gusto. Emotion flooded through me as I enjoyed our special May evening – another memory locked away in the vault for me and vanished for Mum. But this is why it was so important to keep doing it.

Dad turned 80 in May but didn't want a party. He hates being the centre of attention and doesn't like surprises. However, it turned out Mum had emailed friends and invited them to come over, organised a cake and sandwiches, and arranged an 'open house' – all without Dad's knowledge. She'd asked me to help her and I was very torn between wanting to help and knowing that he doesn't really like surprises. However, the emails had already gone out, and the big day arrived.

I went to the shop to pick up the cake, only to find that Dad had already collected it! On the morning of his birthday, Mum had told him what was happening, and as he wasn't sure if she'd organised something or just thought she had, he had gone to the shop to see if there really was a cake for him.

Fresh crab sandwiches were delivered – his favourite – and a steady stream of people came in all day. Dad was so proud of Mum for having pulled it off despite her difficulties, and said he'd had the best birthday ever. It moves me to tears to think back to that day and them both being so happy for one another. Making memories was now becoming a priority for me, and this was exactly the kind of memory I wanted to make.

But the heavy stone was still present. Mum still seemed to think she could drive 'in an emergency' and this worried me silly. Fortunately, though, we are able to laugh at things. Mum has always ordered their wine online and was clearly forgetting she'd ordered a case, so she just ordered another. Dad told me there were 60 bottles of wine stored in the garage. 'Challenge accepted!' I joked (along with the 100 KitKats in the cupboard).

Mum had always been brilliant at managing the family finances, and I made a point of checking every few weeks if she needed help with that. She was absolutely certain that she had it all organised and that there was absolutely nothing to worry about on that front. I worried, but there was also little I could do to force someone who wasn't ready.

Unbeknown to Dad, my sister, and me, May was when Mum had actually begun to stop being able to manage the money. We didn't discover this for months, but we were sitting on a ticking time bomb and the match had been lit.

June

My battery had run flat, so I walked barefoot on the beach, listened to the waves, and tried my hardest to keep the horizon straight. Which is a bit like life.

(Instagram @Seasaltandsarah)

A few friends had suggested I write an article about my wild swimming and send it to *Living Orkney*, the island magazine. It was worth a try, and I scheduled a day to go and visit a friend on the little island of Gramesay. It was a 20-minute boat ride and I could spend the day writing in her home, finish off with a swim in the sea at the end of her garden, and return on the boat. This seemed ideal, so I booked a cheeky day off from work to devote to my time writing and swimming.

Taking the boat and packing food for lunch, I made my way over to the island and my friend's house. She works from home, so we'd agreed to work in separate rooms and come together for lunch. It seemed ideal, and I sat down in her most enviably located home, looking out over to the lighthouse a stone's throw away and Stromness across the water.

I opened up my laptop and began to prepare to launch into my writing when the phone rang. It was Dad. He was just about to drive Mum to the hospital, as she'd noticed her heart was racing and didn't feel well. The one and only day I'd gone to another island, and I'd already missed the boat returning back to the mainland – the next one being several hours away.

I forced myself to keep calm, relax, and try not to worry. I thought about what I could do rather than what I couldn't, so rang ahead to the hospital to warn them that Mum had dementia and Dad was hard of hearing. I gave them as much information as I could and asked them to call me if there was anything I needed to know. At least Mum was going to be in the best place until I could get back.

Not wanting to worry my sister in America, and aware of the time difference, I decided not to message her until I was back on the mainland a few hours later. There was nothing much to tell at that time, and I was mindful how awful it must be to be so far away.

Having done all I could, I continued writing my article, had lunch and a dip, and returned to the mainland on the next available boat. I went straight to the hospital and found them both on the ward where Mum had now been admitted. Whatever heart incident she'd had seemed relatively minor, and she'd been kept in more as a precaution than anything. She agreed to stay – they weren't going to force her – but later she wanted to go home, as she was fine. I knew Dad was worried and wanted her to stay the night, so I persuaded her to stay and wrote a note for her to find, in case she woke in the night and forgot why she was there.

Mum, you are in hospital for one night following a minor heart episode. You have agreed to stay. Dad will come and collect you and take you home in the morning. Everything is fine.

Everything wasn't fine. My stone suddenly became too heavy to lift. It wasn't just the worry of Mum that was weighing heavy, but the combination of a catalogue of things in my family, home, and work, all colliding to make me feel overwhelmed. I fell down a black hole, or at the very least slid and found myself at the bottom, staring up.

All the lovely weather we'd previously been enjoying died a sudden death, and June started off cold and foggy which, day after day, dragged everyone down. As I pulled my coat closer round me one day and moaned with a group of friends, an Orcadian lady in the group, also trying to keep warm, said, 'Sometimes it's just like this. You wait and wait for summer and it doesn't happen, and all of a sudden it's September and you missed it.' I nearly cried on the spot.

As much as I enjoyed cold water swimming, I wanted some warmth on my skin for the rest of the day. I wanted evening swims at sunset. I wanted morning swims at dawn and to enjoy the warmth on my skin just for a while in its rightful time. It wasn't too much to ask. I was feeling cheated of a summer, and it was beginning to affect my mood.

I had a steady stream of family stresses and worries, and work was busy. Mum and Dad were a constant source of worry, and I know they wouldn't want to be. But I was aware there were things that Mum at the time felt she was managing, but in reality wasn't.

Following their holiday in Lanzarote, Mum had come home and immediately booked a cruise for later in the year. For many years, my parents have enjoyed a holiday in March and November, and this year was to be no different. She still had the capability to book it, and before I knew anything about it, the deed was done.

Both my parents have worked all their life and I certainly didn't begrudge them spending the money they had earned, but I had concerns about travel insurance. And when I tried to question Mum about it, I received varying answers. She was pretty certain she had insurance and it was connected to her bank account, but of course she now had a dementia diagnosis and this needed addressing on the policy. Plus Dad was now over 80, another milestone when it comes to ramping up the fees for insuring people.

I was worried their insurance would be invalid – if they even had it! So I finally managed to convince Mum that we needed to address the issue. One of the benefits for Mum is that she is no longer anxious about stuff like that, but I was concerned something could happen and they would end up losing money on the holiday, or being faced with problems and trying to sort them out whilst abroad.

I went over to their house one afternoon to do it, and the weather had picked up, finally giving us a hot day. I was stressed, had a headache, and spent an hour on the phone on my parents' behalf, discussing travel insurance and trying to find something that covered dementia. As I waded my way through the questions, I was eventually given a quote for them and turned to Mum to tell her. She immediately responded with, 'I'm not paying that!' and the whole afternoon went up in a puff of smoke.

It was one of those pivotal moments. Everything took so much energy to organise and explain and plan, and I was close to tears. Mum and Dad were so grateful for everything I was doing and continually told me so, but I was frequently berating myself that no matter what I did, it just wasn't enough.

As each week passed, we seemed to lose another part of her as the sand shifted and sank beneath us. It was stressful when she ordered the same things off the internet – not because having three blouses mattered in the grand scheme of things, but because it represented the loss and change that dementia was bringing. I was grieving Mum, and Mum was grieving herself.

She was becoming less able, and Dad was having to do things he'd never done before. 'It should've been me,' he said, hugging Mum as we finally gave up on the travel insurance for that day.

I returned home from the efforts to organise travel insurance, utterly bereft. We were a strong family, but the order of things was changing so much. That afternoon stays clearly in my mind; I remember what I was wearing and how sunny it was. I remember having a headache, and strangely wishing I had an ice lolly. I remember driving home and crying in the car on the driveway before going in the house.

My car is my safe space and contains all my feelings and thoughts. The 18-mile journey to and from work every day is where I gather my thoughts, talk to God (often out loud), and listen to music or audio books. Often, when I get home from work, I just sit in the car in the dark for a few minutes before going into the house, just to quiet my mind before the 'What's for tea?' kicks into gear. My husband's car is immaculate and empty. Mine is full of swimming gear, a complete and utter mess, but it's my own personal space that contains my thoughts, my fears, my prayers, my tears.

The doctor decided to sign me off work for a couple of weeks to give me some breathing space. 'Something has to give,' she told me compassionately, and it gave me leave to switch off from work worries and just be present in the sadness of it all.

I was an emotional wreck, and spent the first week staring at the wall, but two weeks was enough and enabled me to get my bounce back.

Even though it felt like summer hadn't even started, mid-summer was fast approaching and a group of us had organised to go on a swimming weekend. One of the group organisers, Peter, had a van that could accommodate us all, and people organised to stay in hostels and B&B's. It was something to really look forward to and we needed little in the way of luggage for the weekend, but I packed all my swimsuits so I always had a dry one to wear.

Peter fashioned a line onto the outside of the van and threaded all our costumes along it, so that they would catch the wind and the worst of the water would dry off as we drove along. It looked absolutely hilarious but was a practical solution to a common swimmers' drying problem.

We were to take a boat to the mainland of Scotland and travel down the west coast. It had all been organised by the 'parents' of the group, as we jokingly called them. I'm not an organizer; I'm happy to just be told what to do, as I spend my working life being organized, and in my own time I'm the opposite. I had one job, which was to be at the boat and join the others to await further instruction. But I somehow got my times in a muddle, and arrived to hear my friends asking security how long I had to get there before being turned away. 'She has one minute before we can't let her on.'

'No-one tell my husband this just happened,' I said as I raced on with seconds to spare. He's a piermaster and meticulous about time-keeping, especially with boats. It's a real bugbear of his when people race down to the boat and expect to be accommodated, when they can't get there on time and ropes have to be thrown, and schedules have to be met. So for me to narrowly miss it meant I would never live it down, and neither would he.

We all gathered in the restaurant to eat tea and sail across to the mainland on the hour-and-a-half crossing. The sea was flat calm and it was a beautiful sailing, but it's not always like that. I've also been on very rough crossings where we've bobbed about like a cork, and while I've lain flat and focused on deep breathing to not throw up I've heard piles of plates smashing as they went flying in the crew galley. Island life is like no other.

In order to break up the journey, we stopped off for a swim at Melvich – a beautiful sandy beach with crashing waves and water so brown and peaty it was like swimming in beer. The sea was warmer by June, enabling us to stay in for longer and lark about in the warm evening sun before continuing on with our journey. We had a second planned swim at solstice sunset, so needed to be at our destination in good time to get ourselves sorted out.

A couple of other swimmers were travelling up to join us as well, and as we drove through the Highlands I drank in the incredible rugged scenery with its stunning waters everywhere I looked.

I was dropped off at my B&B to settle in and met the host. 'I have a dog, and children,' she said with an apologetic warning. 'So do I,' I laughingly replied. Apparently, it was enough to turn some people away, but I'm not that easily deterred.

In Orkney, it doesn't really get dark at all in June, and the same could be said for the Highlands. Our chosen solstice swim spot was at Balnakeil – another beautiful location, which was crowded with many people who had turned out to see the sun set on the longest day. We watched from the waves as the sun disappeared but still left enough light to see our way clearly back to the van. And while some of the group were keen to go on to a third swim, most of us were tired and ready to go to our beds. I was dropped off again at my dog-and-children B&B, and sank into bed exhausted, not expecting to be kept awake with the worst case of after-drop I've ever known.

After-drop is the body's natural response to what you're subjecting it to, when swimming in cold water. As you enter the water, you are putting your body under slight stress, releasing endorphins and causing blood to rush to your core to keep it warm. Your body shuts down the circulation to your skin, and your warm blood is drawn away to your core. When you leave the water and start to warm up, this process goes into reverse. Your blood is recirculated back, and your temperature actually drops a few degrees in the process, so you end up colder than when you were in the water. Drying, dressing, and putting on layers quickly is vital. Covering your head also makes a huge difference, even if you only put a hat on when getting out. A flask of hot drink works wonders, too, and I've more recently discovered the value of wrapping your towel or clothes around a hot water bottle.

After the solstice swim, my routine had been rather slapdash. I didn't take a flask, knowing I would be dropped back at the B&B pretty soon after the swim, and

I just dried and got back in the van in a towel robe with my change robe over the top. Layers are key to warming up, and I didn't take a hat. Nor did I move around very much to warm up.

When I returned to the B&B, I had a shower and put on my pyjamas, had a drink, and went to bed. I don't often shower after a swim; I prefer to warm up more slowly, and showering or hot baths can play a part in feeling unwell and hypothermic after swimming. Probably the combination of minor differences to my usual routine was enough to make my core temperature lower than usual and the after-drop pretty severe.

I got into bed feeling cold and began to shiver, and couldn't stop. It was crazy! I've swum in much cooler temperatures, and it was officially mid-summer, yet here I was lying in bed with my teeth chattering. As it went on and on, I seriously considered calling the others at the hostel down the road and asking for help. I never normally go to bed straight after a swim, and I wonder not enough moving around to warm up had played a part, too.

Eventually, I found a spare blanket in the wardrobe and put that over me as another layer. I must have stopped shivering and fallen asleep in the end, as I was fine by the morning, but it served as a timely reminder to respect the water and its cold all year round.

The weekend was wonderful and a great way to restore me after a painful few weeks. We walked miles to the most incredible beach called Sandwood Bay. It hosts enormous sand dunes, which are exhausting to climb, and crashing waves, one of which took me right off my feet. No fear of after-drop this time, as the sun was boiling that day and the four-mile walk back to the van kept my core cosy.

We stopped off on the way back to our digs for another swim, and had a refreshing dip at another beautiful beach. 'Here be mermaids' said a sign on the gate to the beach steps. Ain't that the truth!

It was at this beach that I encountered my first jellyfish sting. Jellyfish are, without a doubt, the worst part of sea swimming in the summer. The price we pay for warmer water is a varied selection of jellyfish – some harmless, and others not so. Through the summer I was stung about five or six times, but most of them were not bad; it just felt like I'd trodden on a stinging nettle. I didn't even notice at first, because of the cold water, but when I got out and started to warm up, the sting began to hurt. The worst was from a lion's mane, and on that occasion my knee began to hurt as I was driving home. It was so painful I actually pulled over the car to see what was wrong, and saw the tiniest little cut with a bit of red around it. By next morning, it was swollen, bruised, and sore for the whole week. I still have a scar.

So, when jellyfish season arrives, it takes the fun out of wild swimming a bit because you're constantly on the lookout. I remember going in with someone once who was really scared of them, following a nasty sting the previous year. She got in and swam off, and as soon as I looked down, I saw a massive one. I had to keep my cool so as not to alarm her, but really didn't enjoy the swim as I knew it was lurking somewhere. Also, before you ask, peeing on jellyfish stings is a complete myth. Don't waste your time asking a friend to do the deed. You'll lose a friend and be grossed out all for nothing.

After two or three swims on the Sunday morning, it was time to make our way back towards the Scrabster boat, complete with lots of fun and laughter in the van. We were tired but had thoroughly enjoyed our memorable weekend. As we drove, we kept our eyes on the coast all the time in case there was a suitable place to dip, but not wanting to miss the boat either.

'How far is it on the map?'

'Three squares.'

'Chocolate comes in squares, not distance!'

I was no longer allowed to be in charge of the map, but I was restored.

July

'I've forgotten your husband's name,' said my mum apologetically mid-conversation, and I thought I might choke and die on the lump in my throat. Then the conversation moved on and she was as right as rain, talking about her childhood and nursing career. 'I've had a lovely afternoon,' she told me as I dropped her home. That's good. So have I.

(Diary entry after an afternoon out to a tea shop)

Several years ago, I worked as a carer looking after elderly people in their home. Many of them had dementia struggles, and they lived alone or with a spouse or family coming in. I went on a six-week training course to help me learn all about dementia, and absolutely loved my job. I was in my element communicating with elderly people, and had a special interest in dementia.

One charming elderly man lived with his wife and had family support from his children. I had such a good relationship with him and his wife that I was asked to continue privately when I changed jobs. This was something I was delighted to do and went to visit him on a weekly basis where we would take walks, or I would read to him from one of his many books. A very well read and learned man, he struggled to express himself verbally, but understood well. We had a beautiful relationship and I grew to love him as a grandfather-type. He reaped what he sowed in terms of having a loving and supportive family around him, and I was always made to feel welcome and part of the gang. His smile lit up the room when you walked in, and his gentle and kindly nature was in the brickwork of his home. I didn't ever know him before his dementia, but I had a strong sense of his character and humour. I was remarking on this in an exchange to his son one evening.

'He's still in there somewhere,' the son said fondly. And I have never forgotten those five words.

Despite all my experience of working with people with dementia, and despite my compassion and understanding, it's different when it's your own family. In my work I hadn't appreciated how I could walk away and forget about it in the evening. I didn't have the million-and-one worries to contend with. I didn't have to watch a seismic shift in a marriage, where husband and wife became carer and cared-for, and how difficult that must be. Nor did I have to see my own role change from daughter to parent of my parent.

I was emotionally involved this time and it was painful, but I was able to draw on my knowledge, experience, and those poignant words, 'She's still in there somewhere.' Mum had by no means disappeared completely; at times she was completely able to focus and be like her former self. But the original clarity was becoming blurred. She was moving out of focus, and no amount of twiddling with the lens could bring back the sharp, high definition woman that had once been there.

Once in a while she would show us the woman she once was, which was wonderful. She regularly had the children in stitches with her remarks, and was like Maggie Smith in *Downton Abbey* when she wanted to make a point.

'I'm not a rabbit!' she told me dryly, rolling her eyes as she pushed a scrap of lettuce away from her favourite crab sandwich in a cafe.

'Aren't you all pessimists!' she once exclaimed in indignation. 'I'm the eternal optimist.'

'I'm not surprised you feel unwell with that ring in your nose, Katie. At least you're not tethered!' She calmly told her granddaughter when she came to visit her in hospital when unwell.

Oh, she was definitely still in there somewhere.

★

Swimming was going swimmingly (I'm not even sorry for that pun). We were now spending much longer in the water as it was so much warmer, occasionally reaching the dizzy heights of 15 degrees. I was falling in love with the underwater world and had a snorkel mask to take a closer look. It made me look like wild swimming meets *Silence of the Lambs,* but it enabled me to see many crabs, sometimes fish, and the biggest starfish I've ever known.

I was now in possession of a *GoPro* – a camera that can be used in the water – and I loved capturing life under the waves as well as above. My daughter suggested I set up an Instagram account devoted entirely to my sea swimming. 'Because it's taking over, Mum,' she told me. So, @seasaltandsarah was born. From this account, I was able to connect with an enormous community of wild swimmers all over the world, with people who had the same passion as I did. As much as I loathe the word 'followers', people were clicking to follow the account, and seemingly enjoying an endless supply of swimming selfies and pictures of Orkney's seas.

Through Instagram and my blog, I now chat to people all over the world, and have made many friends through the internet. I also shared aspects of life with a parent with dementia, and found lots of people messaging to say how much they appreciated it because they were struggling too, or had, and it made them feel connected to others. We were united in living grief, and it cemented my thoughts about writing a book. People clearly wanted to connect over these topics.

My daily dose of 'vitamin sea' was doing me the power of good, and as much as I enjoyed swimming, I also loved larking around in the sea. A few months before, I had seen a picture on Instagram of a woman about the same size as me posing on her back in the water, arms and legs out like a starfish. She'd been photographed by a drone flying above her, and I absolutely loved this image and everything about it. Her confidence and ability to do it was infectious and was something I aspired to.

Since seeing it, I'd wanted to recreate the photo, and banged on about starfishing many times. We finally had an opportunity to make it happen when my friend Ally agreed to stand on the side of the pier and be my personal paparazzi while I struck the pose. It was harder than it looked, and resulted in several hilarious outtakes as I sank in the middle, ended up with my head underwater, and got myself a mammoth ice cream headache. But eventually, thanks to dedication and much laughing, we got the shot and I shared it on my social media pages to raise a smile.

It was liberating for me and showed the transformation taking place, as never in a million years would I have allowed a full body shot to be shown of me before, never mind in a swimsuit pulling a ridiculous pose. But here I was, willingly sharing it and not caring. I was hoping not to test the theory out on my kids that it's possible to actually die of embarrassment, but they both maintained a dignified silence on the matter and are thankfully still here. So seemingly not.

A few weeks later, Ally's husband showed up on the beach with a drone and we did a double starfish, this time looking far more professional. It was such fun, and I loved the pictures. When I later received a necklace from Ally of a starfish cast from one we'd found, it was extra special and had so much meaning to me.

One of the real beauties of the summer months is endless opportunities to swim and have fun in the water. All the extra daylight was the best backdrop to be able to pop down to the sea after tea, before work, or at a 10pm sunset, chatting and laughing in the water as if we were in some kind of group therapy. So much fun was being had in the waves that more than once I took my eye off the ball and ended up running out of the sea to rescue my change robe before the tide took it. It's even been left with a tide mark on it, when I wasn't quite quick enough on one occasion. Swimming in the sea is hard; running in the sea is harder.

The month ended on a high when I took part in my first ever official swimming event. And I use that term loosely. It was the Stromness shopping week – an annual celebration that was started after the war to encourage people to come to the fishing town of Stromness and spend time in the local shops. Loads of events take place for all ages, and it lasts the whole week. One of the events is the Holm's race, where you are taken out to an island in a boat and swim back to the harbour. Distance-wise it's not far – about 16 lengths of the pool – and there are support vessels in case you get tired.

The race was a bit like the equivalent of a fun run for swimmers, and there were three categories: fast, medium, and fun – not slow. I placed myself firmly in the fun category and really wasn't bothered if I finished last. I just wanted to take part and say I'd done it.

What follows is my social media summary for the event.

UNFLUENCER! I took part in my first ever official swimming event today. I use that term loosely. It's the Stromness shopping week Holms race, where you get taken out to an island in a boat and swim back to the harbour.

1. No-one told me I'd have to climb over the side of the boat looking like a beached effing whale and drop into the water in front of all the whizzy fast people in their fancy wetsuits. MOR-TI-FIED.
2. I wore a swimming cap with a local restaurant's name on, so basically I'm now a sponsored athlete – sponsored by food and drink.
3. I came fourth from last; I was just lucky to come in unassisted by the rescue boats around. Shame kept me going.
4. I got stung on my butt by a jellyfish. My husband said it stung as it overtook me.
5. I stuck the GoPro down the front of my cossie to get some underwater action. Only it was the wrong way round and I filmed my cleavage for several minutes before I realised. Footage never to be released.
6. The first picture was taken last night in 'training' – ahahaha, training my ask. I included it

because it's the only one where I don't look like
I fell headfirst out the ugly tree.

All joking apart, I really enjoyed that Holmes race. A friend, Paul, swam alongside me, even though I know he could have swum faster. We chatted and took in the view of Stromness from a completely different angle. There were many ahead of us and a few behind us, but everyone was in brilliant spirits. As one older lady struggled with her footing getting into the water, she exclaimed, 'We can swim, we just cannae walk!' And we all burst out laughing.

Approaching the harbour, there were people clapping and cheering us on as we finished the swim. Even though I frequently swam double that distance in the pool, I was tired. Swimming in sea water, I find, is harder. You have wave resistance, tidal pulls, and cold to contend with, not to mention weather and wildlife. In fact, as we swam, we noticed there was a tidal pull we had to push through in one spot.

Just as we were approaching the very end, I saw a huge jellyfish we were heading straight for. I stopped and trod water, warning Paul, and he swam round it. I warned the others behind me, too, so they knew to avoid it, and went on to finish, walking up the pier steps just behind Paul.

My hugely competitive friend was at the top of the steps to greet me, saying, 'You stopped! And then the man beat you!' She couldn't believe I would let anyone go in ahead of me if I had the chance to be in front.

'He was only behind me because he slowed right down to swim alongside me. If we were really competing, he'd be way ahead of me,' I replied. I was happy to let him go in ahead of me; he thoroughly deserved it. I was just delighted to have completed the event, and I celebrated my achievement with a once-a-year treat of candy floss.

Summer was finally here, and even though it was short, it was enough to restore us for a few weeks as we enjoyed long days, washing pegged on the line, heating switched off, and that feeling of being invincible that summer brings.

I was continuing to try new experiences, but nothing matched the swimming, which I'd undertaken really early on and had completely sidetracked me. I was back at work and working long hours, which meant I often didn't get to daytime swims that were organized, and my FOMO (Fear Of Missing Out) was strong.

Many of the retired people or those with different work patterns planned 'swim adventures'. This was a chance to travel around the island, swimming in a few locations throughout the day. It's amazing the bucket lists that grow for sea swimmers. I'd wanted to swim in the North Sea and Atlantic on the same day.

We achieved this one weekend by driving to one of the barriers and swimming in the North Sea, before crossing over the road to the other side of the barrier and hopping into the Atlantic. ('Why are you bothering? They both splash cold,' said an often bemused Roy.) It was all brilliant fun and brought a great sense of micro adventures to an otherwise ordinary Saturday.

I was squeezing life out of everything I could, and the salt water made my often heavy stone weightless. Maybe this was why I wanted to spend so much time in it.

I was disappointed not to get to one of Lucy's planned adventure days. She was the one who dedicated her swims, and introduced me to that idea in the very beginning. Lucy told me that she sometimes 'swims in the place of...', which I really liked the idea of. So, although I couldn't go, it was touching to know someone was going in my place.

'You had a wonderful time swimming around Barrier One today,' Lucy told me. This time the stone was a tiny lump in my throat, as I found this incredibly moving. The daisy chain of people's small acts of kindness was sustaining me, and as Dad relayed stories of people doing things to support them, it was sustaining him, too.

August

Fun times in giant rock pools today. Getting in and out was incredibly slippery with seaweed, and the most unflattering I've ever been in my entire life. Let's never speak of this again.

(Instagram @seasaltandsarah)

Wild swimming is, without a doubt, the best activity I've ever undertaken, but comes with an unfortunate side-effect. Getting dressed. The getting dressed routine is the most nightmarish hell on earth, especially if it's windy or, worse, still raining. I'm finally coming to terms with it and don't mind so much now, but the first 250 times were the worst.

Men have it so much easier, as they can just dry their top half with freedom and abandon then get their layers on quick. Women, on the other hand, have to wrestle with taking a wet top half off and getting a dry top half on, all without revealing side boob – and it's no easy feat! Salt water is sticky, and you try pulling a top over yourself that's rolled itself up at the back, all as it's blowing a gale and sending a wind chill right through you enough to freeze your organs.

I made numerous attempts to master the dark art and streamline my getting dressed routine, all very badly. Some people dress in the back of their car, but that never appealed to me – 'besides, space is an issue; I already told you it's a permanent mess, there's never any room in the back of my car; it's so full of miscellaneous crap. Added to this, there's a cosmic law that says you could be on a deserted beach/car park for 15 hours, but dog walkers will appear just as you are pulling off your costume.

In a desperate attempt at some vague kind of modesty, I scoured the internet for a pop-up changing tent, and found one for less than twenty quid. I chose bright pink, and it caused much hilarity. It was quickly named my 'pink tardis', and sceptics in the group said it would be zero use on a windy day (correct). But in the summer, when car parks are often full of campervans and people eating their breakfast outside, it was a necessary item and meant I could dress and head off to work with my modesty (and side boob!) intact.

I've heard sniggering, too, while dressing, but I'd rather be laughed at for that than flashing my backside. Change-robes sell themselves for getting dressed under, but in reality it's not that easy getting dressed underneath one. It is, though, handy for throwing over yourself, zipping up, and taking a wet costume off, whilst keeping warm and modest.

A group of us once went to a secluded beach and had our swim. Just as we were all pulling our costumes down, wriggling about under our change-robes, a coach party arrived filled with what felt like a thousand people. Unbelievable timing! So, we sweltered in heavy change-robes and headed up the 60 or so steps to the car and my trusty tardis.

I'll let you in on a secret: wild swimmers often drive home 'commando', as faffing about with bras and knickers wastes valuable time. So, we often pick elasticated waist trousers and baggy tops to throw on, and get our layers on as quickly as we can. I'm straying into too much information territory now, but I tend to put easy pull-on knickers on, and a friend once asked me why I bothered.

'I don't want to be knickerless, just in case I get stopped by the police,' I told her.

'Are they likely to ask you to pull your trousers down?' she laughingly asked. I guess she had a point.

August was the thing of dreams for wild swimmers. Although I didn't get quite the same cold water buzz that cooler months gave me, I was certainly able to enjoy plentiful swimming opportunities, nipping down to the beach after tea in the evening, or venturing a little further and being in the water for a glorious sunset.

One Friday a group of us met up at Evie beach and swam, followed by a bonfire and campfire food. Peter brought dough and we cooked bread on hot stones, ate sausages, and toasted marshmallows, washed down with hot chocolate or even a beer for some. The usual laughter and in-jokes took place before the tide came and washed away the last of the campfire embers, but not the memories.

Another gloriously hot Saturday afternoon was spent at 'Amy's Pools'. In her book *The Outrun,* Amy talks about huge rock pools at the end of the farm where she grew up. As she was up visiting family and it was a chance to meet up, she arranged a swim there – and it was the best of afternoons. At low tide you can access the rock pools, jump off rocks into the water, and children could climb and play on the giant slabs of rock warming up in the sun. More sausages, more marshmallows, and the ambiance of a lazy summer day that could go on forever.

Getting into the rock pools was easy; you just sat on the side and dropped in. Getting out was much harder, as the edges of the multiple pools were covered in slippery seaweed. It was handy to hold onto and pull yourself up, but probably pretty traumatising for the people behind me, seeing me crawl out on my hands and knees (Sorry, Mim, I know you were one!). You swam and climbed through a series of rock pools and eventually arrived at the open sea, where for once it was just for looking, not swimming. The force of the waves as they swirled and looked for places to fill over the rocks, created quite a pull that I had no desire to be dragged out by.

'Water's always in such a hurry to find somewhere to go,' my husband once told me. And you only have to observe swirling water at cliffs and rock faces to know what he means.

This particular Saturday was idyllic, and the waters kind. But as we sat around on hot slabs of stone, eating our BBQ, we heard stories of when it had been less so. One occasion when the seas had been wild and fierce in winter, a baby seal had been washed right over the top of the giant rocks and into the neighbouring field, where the famer dragged it back into the sea – probably more than a little worse for wear after its ordeal.

By now the lowest temperature I'd swum in was 3.8 degrees and the highest is 15 degrees. Many times I've heard people say things about the sea temperature not really changing much in Orkney waters, but having tried and tested this, I can assure you this belief is entirely untrue.

When I was on holiday, Roy got talking to a man on another table at dinner and told him about my sea swimming. 'Ah well, it's easy, you've got that warm gulf up there,' the man told me with his powerful wisdom and manly views. It was as though I was somehow threatening his masculinity by having a hobby that took a bit of grit to get in, and therefore he had to minimise it. So, I invited him to join me in the alleged warm gulf he spoke about – a warm gulf of six degrees – and the conversation quickly ended.

As well as swimming, the summer months lend themselves to seeing all sorts of tourist attractions in Orkney. Every day, I drive past the Ring O' Brodgar – a Neolithic stone circle which predates Stonehenge. People come from far and wide to visit all the ancient and unspoiled monuments all over Orkney, and I get to see them every day.

The sun rises over the stones, so as I travel to and from work, I often stop and take pictures for friends on social media who don't get to enjoy them as I do. I also drive past other local standing stones (Stenness) and Maeshowe – an ancient chamber, later invaded by Norse crusaders, and which hosts some fine runic graffiti akin to modern-day wisdom, like 'I am very tall and can reach up here' and 'For a good time, call Betty.'

The entrance to the chamber is aligned so the midwinter setting sun shines right in the doorway and lights up the chamber. Our ancestors were a clever bunch. On my daily commute, I continually realise how fortunate I am living here and to be able to access these places that many come to for a once-in-a-lifetime viewing.

One thing I've not been so lucky in seeing in my whole time in Orkney are orcas. During summer months there are often sightings which people post on Facebook. Pods came right into the harbour several times, as groups tried to rescue them and herd them back out to sea. But despite numerous notifications saying where they were, by the time I finished work to go for a look, they had gone.

I once spent the entire summer in Orkney, only leaving the island for a week to visit my daughter in London. During that week away, orcas came right into the shore at Skaill beach, a stone's throw from my house, and people were able to stand on the shoreline and film them. I missed the whole thing, and was hugely disappointed. I have always seemed to be in the wrong place at the wrong time, but maybe it's not a bad thing when I'm swimming. If I saw one when I was in the sea, I'm sure I'd be out of the water like a shot.

Something else was always in a hurry besides the sea, and that was Mum's advancing dementia. The relentless waves were coming in faster than anyone had ever dared believe. Micro changes were revealing themselves on what felt like a daily basis and, rather like the butterfly effect, some seemingly innocuous event in the grand scheme of things represented another shift in the sand beneath us. For example, Mum offering to make drinks for everyone then returning to ask where she kept the coffee. So tiny, yet so huge, showing how things were changing.

What I find so fascinating about the human mind is the ability to 'forget', or rather 'not process', things as basic as where a coffee jar is stored. How many cups of coffee had Mum made in that house over the last ten years? How many times had she boiled the kettle, reached into the cupboard above, and pulled out a coffee jar? Three times a day over ten years would amount to 10,950 times. So why does the autopilot fail at 10951? Why does the brain not assume the obvious – that the coffee lives above the kettle? Boil kettle, reach up hand to cupboard above, make coffee, repeat.

Mum has always been extremely organized. So much so that if I hadn't been born at home I'd swear she had taken the wrong baby back from the hospital. I'm creative – sub text: disorganised. It would be entirely normal for me to not remember where I put something, and it happens on a daily basis. Not so for Mum.

Dad was taking on increasing amounts of responsibilities in the house, and my sister and I were doing all we could to support him, even if it was just emotionally. Mum has always been a very strong woman and is still strong now, but at the same time something was missing. She was now sleeping much later and for longer. I'm sure trying to navigate your way through an ever more bewildering world is exhausting, so I can fully sympathise with her.

She was still able to hold a conversation very well, and this is where it can be tricky to the outside world who think everything is fine and maybe Mum was 'not that bad'. The difficulty came with Mum remembering she'd had the conversation once it was over. The phone call had ended, the person had walked away, and it was hit or miss if Mum remembered having spoken.

Dementia is a well-worn path that many have walked before and, drawing from their experiences, I was always trying to keep my finger on the pulse of how we could manage. The uncertainty of the future is always difficult to navigate, but I was keen to have systems in place to minimise negative impact, if needed. Mum wasn't wandering off, but other people have, completely randomly and without warning. What could I do as a 'just in case'?

I found online a medic-alert bracelet which Mum agreed to wear, and it gave me peace of mind that should she end up somewhere confused, someone could look at her bracelet and find out her condition, name, date of birth, and my phone number. Remarkably, she puts it on every single day without fail and without having to be reminded by Dad. Hopefully, it'll never be needed, but it gave us reassurance as we desperately tried to fight the incoming tide with whatever barriers we could.

It was the middle of August when I came across an initiative run by Alzheimer's Research UK, called Swimming Down Dementia. This was an opportunity to do a sponsored swim over September and October, to raise money for research into Alzheimers and dementia. A friend and swimming companion had signed up to do it, which is how I became aware of the opportunity, and it took me two seconds to make the decision to take part. It was a combination of two things that were so vitally important to me, and an opportunity to hopefully make a difference and do something positive from such a difficult diagnosis.

I set up a fund-raising page and knew I had reach through my blog and other social media platforms. So, I wrote a small piece about what I was aiming to do in the coming months, which was to swim 20 miles in the sea and pool, and shared my donations page, asking people to give a little something towards it. I even offered to dedicate a swim to someone or in memory of someone, and share pictures of the swim.

I set the page up at around 6pm one evening, and by 7pm I had raised £200; £350 by bedtime! It was remarkable. As the money just poured in, I was greatly humbled by the generosity of so many. By the following morning, the money raised had gone up to £500 and it was jaw-dropping. The whole thing didn't even start for another two weeks, and every time I set a new target, it was smashed by the generosity of others.

Roy and I were so moved by this that he said if I could reach £1000 before the whole thing started in September, he would do the challenge, too. I think he had every confidence I would, and I hit the £1k with several days to spare. It was incredibly touching and a great way of dealing with the feeling of helplessness that comes with dementia – in some way I was helping.

I was thankful for the opportunity, and approached a couple of companies to see if they would like to support me in some way. A few gave me products and freebies, including Smoc Smoc who gave me a loose towelling change-robe, and all my changing hell was resolved just like that. If only the rest of life was that easy.

September

Still holding hands after 55 years. On their wedding day they had no clue what lay ahead of them, but they have ridden the storms of multiple cancer, heart bypass, and the loss of a son. Now they are dealing with Mum's declining memory due to dementia, and haven't let go of each other. Dementia is such a painful disease to watch play out. It's a privilege to see them approach this devastating blow with such courage.

(Norq from Ork an Orkney Writer Facebook page)

In a bedroom in Kettering in 1942, a baby girl was delivered into the world. She was named Elisabeth Florence Saile, and her arrival brought much joy to her parents, aunt, and grandparents living next door. In those days, mothers were instructed to take bed rest for the first few weeks after giving birth, and Elisabeth's mother, Mary, did this. She developed a blood clot and died when Elisabeth was just around five weeks old, leaving a family devastated, and a baby without a mother to raise her.

Her Aunt Ella stepped in and raised her while her father worked, and she knew the adoring love of her father, aunt, and grandparents for many years. By the time she was ten, Elisabeth was volunteering at the local hospital and knew she wanted to be a nurse. Nursing was all she ever wanted to do, and she was absolutely brilliant at it. Elisabeth, later named Liz, went away to study nursing in the days when Matron was never questioned, and specialised in paediatric nursing at Birmingham Children's Hospital. It was while living in Birmingham that Liz met Colin, and they went on to have three children – Ann, Simon, and Sarah. Elisabeth is my mum.

I often wonder if it was the loss of her own mother in such devastating circumstances that caused her to have such a vocation and desire to nurse others, or if she would have taken that path anyway.

Mum has always loved nursing, and my entire childhood is filled to brimming with memories of her and hospital life. In those days, the uniform was a dress and belt with a silver buckle. White, removable cuffs on the sleeves, and a hat that was firmly secured into place by two grips. The pristine uniform was all worn under a long cape that buttoned at the neck. Capes weren't just for superheroes – they were also for nurses, like my mum.

I could tell you a million stories of mum's endless patience and care as a nurse. Once a nurse always a nurse. And when she progressed to Ward Sister, she ran a tight ship. Her compassion and kindness for the sick and vulnerable knew no limits, and whilst enjoying paediatrics she also thoroughly enjoyed working in Accident and Emergency, theatres as a scrub nurse, and Birmingham Skin Hospital, from where my short but favourite story derives.

Birmingham Skin Hospital no longer exists as a stand-alone hospital, but in its time it was a small hospital of two wards – one for men and one for women. Mum worked there in the 80s as a bank nurse, and found a real interest in the field. 'If people need to be hospitalised for their skin conditions, then it's bad,' she told me. And even now she can often be moved to tears at the plight of people with terrible skin diseases.

She heard countless stories from her patients about society's rejection of people with such visible illness. People would rather stand than sit next to them on the empty seat on a bus. One man said the quickest way to clear a space on the beach was for him to lay his towel out and undress to his swimming trunks, revealing his flaking dry skin. People were simply repulsed. And I can even recall when my daughter had eczema on her hands as a little girl in primary school, children refusing to hold her hand for a game, and how hurtful it was. Multiply that by a body covered in skin disease and you can begin to imagine how difficult it must be, without even starting on the pain and itching.

Mum eventually became Ward Sister of the men's ward, and instructed all the nurses and staff in a practice she insisted on. 'When a patient arrives on the ward, the first thing you must do before anything else is extend your hand toward them and shake theirs as a welcome. It's vital that they feel accepted and valued, regardless of their appearance.'

This story still chokes me, and makes me feel so proud, over 30 years later. This small simple act would serve to reassure many on their arrival to the hospital, and no-one would be made to feel repulsive or unsightly. At least, not on her watch.

One of my favourite photos of Mum and Dad is one taken of them on their wedding day. It was a candid photo, completely unplanned and unposed. They are standing outside the church, and Dad is holding Mum's hand and she has her head back and is laughing. They are full of marital joy and hope, vows just made, cake not yet cut. No idea they would have three children; no idea one of those children would die before them; no idea Mum would face cancer twice, back surgery, feet surgery; and Dad heart surgery. No idea that over 50 years after this photo was taken, they would still be holding hands and navigating their way through the rocky waters of dementia.

The photo carries such poignancy for me. The transition from a young married couple to an old married couple has happened over 55 years of knowing all the ways and rituals of each other. One starting a sentence, the other finishing it. Each knowing just how the other likes their coffee, each knowing where the coffee jar is.

When my brother died in 2008, I grieved for the loss of a brother and I grieved for my parents' loss of a son. I don't know which was more painful; it would shift and change on an hour by hour basis. My loss, their loss, their loss, my loss. When Mum was diagnosed with dementia, I grieved for the loss of my mother, I grieved for my dad's loss of his wife, and I grieved for my mum's loss of herself. Although Mum was still in there, and in many ways still very much herself, there was so much loss.

Grief isn't about a person dying, grief is about loss.

Read that again.

I remember when my son Elliot left home a few months before mum's diagnosis. My grief was overwhelming and all-consuming. My empty nest was like an echo chamber, and the pain of him going was almost physical. I cried so much prior to him leaving that I once had to pull over the car and be sick at the side of the road. It was important to let him go and for him not to feel inhibited by his sobbing mother clinging onto him, and I knew I had to get it together and do my crying in private. It was the same with Mum and Dad. I didn't want them to see me crying and distressed; they had enough on their plate. I've done a lot of crying in cars.

September is never an easy month for me, as I can struggle with the season shift and the anticipation of the dark nights drawing in. I was beginning to feel anxious about swimming opportunities being diminished due to the lack of light, and no longer being able to swim before and after work.

As I drove home from Mum and Dad's one evening, I was so heavy-hearted I wondered about stopping off for a swim to reset me, but the light was beginning to fade. I drove to the swim spot and sat looking out at the sea, wondering if I would go in, but eventually made the decision not to. Voting in favour of safety, I drove away, still heavy-hearted. I've discussed with others that sometimes the decision on arrival not to swim is a swim. This may not make sense to you, but it does to us. It's all part of the journey. Turning your back on a swim isn't an easy one, but can be a right one in the bigger picture of sea swimming life.

By 1st September, when my Swimming Down Dementia officially started, I had already raised £1300. For my first swim, a group of people wanted to be involved, and as it fell on a Sunday, we were blessed with time and a decent day. A lady turned up who had heard of my fundraising and took part in her first cold water swim. Her own mother had died of dementia the year before, and she swam, donated, and gave me a beautiful bracelet to sell and donate the proceeds to the cause. She also went on to thoroughly enjoy cold water swimming, and has since done it on a regular basis.

Others came along in support, and even brought inflatable flamingos. We posed in the sea for the all-important selfie, which involved Roy climbing onto a buoy to get us all in. It's no easy feat in the sea and I still don't know how he managed it, but I was just happy to have him swimming with me. Roy made a valiant effort to do the 20 miles with me, but unfortunately he has considerable health problems of his own, and eventually I banged the gavel and said enough was enough. No-one was going to ask for their money back if he didn't complete the challenge, and I would complete it on behalf of both of us. Reluctantly, he pulled out after several weeks.

As well as Mum and Dad having their wedding anniversary in September, Roy and I also celebrated ours. Dad has always been a great dancer, so natural and easy. And whilst we used to die of embarrassment as kids, now we were proud to see our parents take to the dance floor and jive. On our wedding day, they jived, and Fiona managed to get a video of them. She shared it on Facebook, and it was enormously well received.

A friend told me only recently that it was the highlight of our wedding day when Mum and Dad took to the dance floor and astounded everybody with their moves. 'Everyone watched this old couple walk onto the dance floor, and then everyone cleared out of the way as they just danced like a boss!' she told me. 'It was absolutely brilliant!'

Mum and Dad have since hung up their dancing shoes, but I will always be grateful to Fiona for capturing that moment, and it comes up on my Facebook memories every year. I'm just sad that Fiona is no longer here to share the memory with.

As much as I struggle with this particular season change, I absolutely love seeing the fields after harvest. The light is an exquisite backdrop to fields full of hay bales for a couple of weeks, and represents in a really physical way the ever-changing seasons, both in a physical sense of the year but also in our lives.

The simplest of phrases has taken me through the darkest of days. 'This too shall pass.' I know this is a truth for the season I am currently in. Nothing is forever, including this. The good days move on and so do the bad; it's a constant cycle of seasons. We can be in the midst of winter and enjoy the warmth of summer sun through the simple act of human kindness. Someone offering to visit, help, be at the end of the phone.

I cherish the lucid times with fun and laughter, whilst telling myself, 'She's still in there somewhere' as I temporarily abandon worry and hope that 'It might just work out ok'. And then it metaphorically snows, you sweep the path, and it snows again, and you wait for it to pass.

Fiona, knowing she was terminally ill, had made many of her wishes known about what should happen to her. And she had wanted to be buried on the island of Westray, where she had grown up and loved. A small group of us who had met with Fiona on a weekly basis, were trying to arrange a visit together to go and lay flowers on her grave. Coordinating three working women to get away for a weekend to Westray proved harder than we thought, but finally an opportunity came in September. We hired a small bothy (a little cottage) for the weekend, complete with an original box bed – highly practical for cold nights, I discovered – and made the journey to Westray.

We had gone as a four the year previously, and this weekend was bittersweet with the memories of our time with Fiona then and the fact that she was missing this time. But we were reunited around her grave as we lay our basket of flowers and wrote our cards. We shed tears, read some Bible verses, and offered our prayers of thanks for the time we'd had together, before returning to our weekend bothy to share a gin and tonic and raise a glass to the friend we knew would absolutely approve.

October

Sometimes it's good, sometimes it's gooder. Perfect sunrise, perfect setting, perfect company, perfect everything.

(Instagram @seasaltandsarah)

Every six months, due to one measly hour's time change, my life disappears into a black hole and I wonder if I will ever find my way back out. On the fateful morning, I woke up and checked the time. The clock on my phone says 6.30, but does that mean 5.30, 6.30 or 7.30am? Is it January, October, Summer, Wednesday, Thursday or Friday? What country am I in? Did the phone remember to magically reset itself or do I have to do it? Will I ever remember how to adjust the time on the oven?

'What time is it?' I ask Roy.

'It's 6.30,' he replies.

'So, is it really 5.30 then?'

'Go back to sleep.'

I moan about the clock changing every time. I'm thrown into a fog of confusion for a week over that 60 minutes, and for me, it's hardly worth the bother. I'm exhausted and confused, it's getting dark so early, and I'm depressed.

I wonder if, on a very small scale, this is how it is for Mum. There's certainly confusion over what day it is, and if it's morning or afternoon. Have we eaten? Did I have my meds? Where are we going again? What day is it? Remind me what your surname is again. Where are we going? Where do we keep the cake forks/coffee/coffee/coffee/coffee, remind me where we're going?

Although this book finishes at the end of 2019, the confusion lives on as I continue to write. While we were on holiday in early 2020, Mum was heading to bed on day 5 and asked, 'Did we just arrive today?'

Time vanishes, reappears, speeds up, slows down. Time brings confusion instead of rhythm and order. And whatever the concept of time, I know I don't have enough of it. Not enough to fit in everything I want to and need to, and not enough to cram in all the memories before the sands run out.

My day starts early as I head off for a swim before work, then it's work, and lunchtime where I shop for food, pay bills, buy birthday cards, and go back to work. On my way home, I stop off to buy the things I forgot at lunchtime. I arrive home and light the fire, make the tea, and wait for Roy to come home. We eat together, watch soaps, and fall asleep on the couch. Sometimes I go over to Mum and Dad's to help with mail or something that's troubling them. I don't mind doing this and don't resent it; I just don't have enough time to give them what I would like to.

Time is such a luxury, I've discovered. Little did I know back in October that COVID-19 was going to hit the headlines in just a few months and throw everything into chaos. Little did I know I would be isolating at home and have more time than I've ever known, with nothing to do and nowhere to go. Be careful what you wish for.

But despite complaining that we don't have enough time, I can see that I made time for the things I love, which was outdoor swimming. By now I was much more streamlined about my routine, but a large part of outdoor swimming seems to be devoted to faffing. I can see many other wild swimmers nodding sagely as they read about faffing, because it's absolutely a thing. You faff about when you arrive, getting your shoes and gloves ready, leaving your towel in a place where it's easy to grab afterwards, setting your clothes out ready to put on in order, then rake about in your bag for the thermometer, camera, and kitchen sink. There are occasional non-faffers but they're a rare breed, because faffing is part of the ritual. Sometimes I faff less, but I never don't faff at all.

The mornings in October were glorious and the sunrises never failed day after day. A few weeks before, the lovely Anna had moved to Orkney. As an outdoor swimmer from before, she was keen to continue in Orkney, always posting sunrise swims she could do to get her up in the morning and ready for the day ahead. Mornings are probably my favourite time to swim, as it gets me up and out of bed, and invigorates me for the day ahead. We often say that if one of us didn't post a swim event, then we would most likely all still be in bed. But group swimming gives us the motivation to keep on going.

I had a week off work but still got up every morning to swim at sunrise with Anna and a few others she had encouraged into the water. It ended up being a memorable week. The colours of the sky as the sun rose gently, the fishing boats going by as they set off for their day's catch, seeing Stromness chug into life against the backdrop of the Hoy hills, and the gentle sound of gulls and lapping water, were all magical. I even managed my first moonlight swim, although – full disclosure – it was just because the moon was still visible in the morning!

On one of those special mornings, there was a group of us swimming as usual, and on this day we were all-female. We'd been in about 20 minutes when a man came long, eyeing up the water and somewhat surprised to see us. He said he was up in Orkney for work and he'd been thinking of going for a dip.

'I figured if you guys are in there, it can't be that bad,' he said with casual sexism. He then made a big display of wowing us all with his impressive jumping off the pier and into the water, before exiting two minutes later, leaving us all desperately trying to keep a straight face. Women can do hard (and cold) things. Just saying.

On my swimming bucket list since my early swimming days had been a swim around the Inganess shipwreck at Hallowe'en. The day was fast approaching and, having never swum in the dark, I had a mix of excitement and nerves. When the day arrived, we all met in the car park at the beach and donned swimming lights and torches for our tow floats. I, of course, was as slapdash as ever and couldn't find a working torch, so grabbed a set of battery-operated fairy lights I could lay my hands on, and shoved that in my dry bag. It had pretty much the same effect and lit up my tow float like a glowing pumpkin.

Seventeen of us went excitedly down to the beach and into the water where the huge shipwreck loomed ahead of us as a giant dark shadow. There were squeals of excitement and chatter as we all hurried around the wreck. In my experience, we always seem to swim anticlockwise; I once swam clockwise with a friend and it felt most peculiar, like working with two left hands, and I've never done it since. As we swam in the dark, the water glistened with phosphorus, which was something I'd never seen before let alone swum in. It was magical and looked like a million stars reflecting off the water. I discovered at this swim that it's also pretty easy dressing in the dark as you don't have to worry quite so much about modesty. Thankfully, no-one can see you. I'm sure in my case that thankfulness is a two-way street.

As with every swim, I drove home with my trusty travel cup of hot chocolate. But this comes with a word of caution. If spilling hot chocolate was a super-power, I'd be your hero. Clad in cape and pants outside my tights, I could save the world from COVID-19 with my unparalleled hot chocolate spilling powers. Alas, it's not, and I can't, but that hasn't stopped me from spilling it a record number of times. Being guilty of a sweet tooth, hot chocolate is my post-swim drink of choice, and that means the flask is very hard to keep clean. So, I made it in a thermal travel cup and took that. However, I've lost count of the number of times I've spilled hot chocolate in my own car and, embarrassingly, in other people's. I once had to mop up the footwell of Ally's van with a hat (hers). And the passenger seat of mine has ambiguous brown stains on it thanks to my setting the cup on the seat and forgetting, causing it to tip over and leak hot brown liquid everywhere when I drive.

I carry my neoprene shoes and gloves in a washing-up bowl, as they are always wet, and have arrived at a swim to find them swimming in hot (now cold) chocolate, thinking it would be a good idea to set the cup in there. I've been extra careful only to have the lid fly off, making the cup fall from under it and the chocolate disperse in 15 different directions. I had a problem I needed solving. I eventually bought a flask which is filled with water, and I take the travel cup with the dry powder and a spoon to make the drink once I'm out of the water. Life is a journey; we are always learning.

★

It turns out there are always projects and challenges to keep swimmers motivated throughout the year, and the

Human Excellence Project organised a global swimrise. People from all over the world swam at their sunrise and shared the photos – some in considerably warmer climates than ours! But having a reason and motivation to get up can sometimes be the make or break of a day, especially if you're feeling low and unmotivated. I've found as my swimming journey continues that challenges both big and small keep me on track. If I hear of something and get the first inkling of a notion that it might be doable in my life, then I simply HAVE to do it. I get on my own nerves sometimes, because I frequently complain I have no time whilst simultaneously signing up for other challenges.

So, it's little surprise that when limited places to swim in the Polar Bear Challenge came up – a chance to swim throughout winter, meeting certain challenges along the way – I was signed up and ready to finish my Swimming Down Dementia on October 31st and start my Polar Bear Challenge on 1st November.

Due to the marriage of a family friend, both children returned home, which was extra special. If there's one downside to living in Orkney, it's the distance from my children Katie and Elliot, the cost of traveling here, and the time taken to get home. Family get-togethers are both rare and extra precious.

I was over the moon to have my brood back in the nest, even for a short while, and considered once again if what happened to mum should happen to me. It saddened me, and them, for them to see their beloved granny sometimes so bewildered. She still knew who they were, and for that, I am so thankful. Each family is unique, each decision complicated. Mercifully, I didn't need to make any decisions other than to remind the children to enjoy every moment with Granny. They both showed enormous compassion, patience, and understanding. They love their grandparents very much, and that's also a two-way street.

The money was pouring in for my sponsored dementia swim, and by the end of the challenge I'd raised just under £3000 with offers and Gift Aid. I was overwhelmed and very humbled at people's generosity. I remained top of the leader board for fundraising for almost the entire duration of the challenge, just being knocked off at the very end. It was the first time I'd been top of a leader board for any sporting event, and I made sure I milked it. The fact it had little to do with sporting prowess was a mere detail.

Nevertheless, I was committed to finishing the challenge, and I tended towards little and often swims, especially as the water was getting colder and I still had a full-time job to manage. My boss was becoming quite used to me sitting in the office with a huge change-robe on, plus a scarf and hot water bottle. Colleagues frequently jibed me for my craziness, and I would frequently tell them not to knock it 'til they tried it, and invite them to join me.

'Why would I want to go in the sea? It's full of plastic straws and nutters like you,' said one.

Fair point.

While swimming at Inganess one morning, I was filming underwater and saw the biggest starfish I've ever laid eyes on. As I pointed my camera at it, the starfish moved one of its legs and it appeared to be waving at me. It reminded me of the beautiful story of the man who saw a boy throwing a starfish back into the sea after thousands had been washed up on the beach. The man questions the boy as to why he is doing it, when there are so many stranded. The boy simply throws a starfish back into the sea and replies, 'It made a difference to that one.'

Sometimes I've been the starfish thrower and made a difference to the one. More often than not, I've been the starfish, and some beautiful person has picked me up and thrown me gently back into the ocean. As my grief snowballed along with my need for a shoulder to cry on, I quietly thanked all those who had helped me when I'd been stranded, and sent it out into the atmosphere.

November

M is for Mum. It was very poignant to finish my swimming down dementia challenge on the same day my magazine article about Mum was published. When I saw it in print, I was unable to read it, it was too moving, even though I was the one who wrote it.

(Instagram @Seasaltandsarah)

In November 2019, I was so full of feelings and emotions about everything that had happened over the last 11 months that I decided it was time to organise myself to write a book. This was something I've wanted to do for a very long time, and it felt like I now had enough material that could be neatly slotted into a year. My book mentor was in place, and I made a little announcement on social media.

The response was enormous, and I was overwhelmed. My imposter syndrome was strong and I felt all manner of emotions about doing it, and had to regularly remind myself that I'd had hundreds of people message me telling me how they felt about me sharing my story and how they were looking forward to the book. This encouragement keeps me going when I struggle.

As I write this now in April 2020, we are in the middle of the COVID-19 crisis and the world has become a scary place. The pool has closed and there's no meeting to swim in groups. In fact, for many outdoor swimmers, the idea of swimming outdoors at all was discouraged because of driving to swim spots, as well as risks that could put the system under increased strain. And the RNLI asked people not to. It was not about us, but about supporting the people who didn't have the luxury of making that choice.

The world has flipped on its head, and we are using language that we'd never even heard of a few weeks previously: social distancing, self-isolating, lockdown. We are playing endless games of Scrabble with total strangers, jumping around breathlessly to celebrities who are hardwired to motivate the planet, breathing in and out to yoga experts offering their relaxed energy to the world, and listening to celebrity singers crooning from their huge houses as their hair gets steadily longer and Botox faces saggier.

Everyone is doing live Instagrams, free online courses, coughing discreetly, sharing their soup recipes, baking with all the leftover ingredients in the house, buying all the toilet paper, pasta, and tins of beans. People are distanced and yet more connected. The world will never be the same again, but we probably said that after the war... both of them.

This is what's happening in real-time, as I write this book. But in November, I was blissfully unaware of what was just around the corner. Temperatures were plummeting and exhilaration rising. Seaweed was dying back and mirroring the gardens above. I can now know for certain that the colder the better when it comes to cold water high.

Roads were icy, and mornings cold and crisp. I was still desperate to fulfil my dream of swimming in ice at some point, and opportunity presented itself a couple of times in November. Driving to work one frosty morning, the sky was lit up a hundred shades of pink and the lochs were frozen. This was my moment; my golden opportunity to step into the ice water and add a tick to my bucket list. But I made a promise to myself that I wouldn't attempt to swim in ice alone, so I drove on past the loch disappointed but knowing I was doing the right thing.

I did, however, manage a swim in the sea on the same day, and after crunching over frosty seaweed I entered the waters to a chilly 4.5 degrees. When alone, I am careful not to go out of my depth and take all precautions necessary to ensure I stay safe. Even in company, I am learning all the time. I once swam to the end of a working pier and back, only to see a small boat head around the pier at a steady speed. It shook me a little, and Roy reminded me that even if I was wearing a hi-vis tow float, boats can't slam their brakes on like a car. I've never done it again.

I once swam around the shipwreck without my tow float, and just as I made it to the shallow waters, two ribs (rigid inflatable boats) from a liner came up at speed to the wreck for a look. They would never have seen me in the water, and once again I was spooked and thankful for the narrow escape, vowing to always wear my tow float from thereon in.

Having ended my dementia swim challenge, I joined with others in starting the Polar Bear challenge, and people participated at varying levels. No-one judged the other for doing more or less towards the challenge, each operating in a way that was suitable for them. I opted for the most basic challenge, which allowed the wearing of gloves and shoes. Having had a really unpleasant experience earlier in the year with numb hands, it just wasn't an option for me to go gloveless and try to fit it around work.

This was also going to be my first swim through winter, and I had no idea how I was going to cope, so I happily joined the 'penguin' category and released any pressure to do or be better. I wasn't competing with anyone, just happy to challenge myself. If you'd told me a year ago that I would be heading for the sea at every given opportunity, I would have said you were mad. But here I was, and my life had changed beyond recognition. I had met many likeminded people on social media, particularly Instagram, and now have an army of friends I've yet to meet.

At last, I was able to achieve one of my bucket list

goals, which was to have a full moon swim. A small group of us met at Ness and headed into the water, which was around seven or eight degrees, and had the most magical swim. The moon shone on the waves and the lights of Stromness were visible across the water. We joked at how an ice cream headache could be achieved in those harder-to-reach areas, and we exited feeling revived and thrilled at our swim.

My sister, Ann, who lives in Colorado, came to visit for ten days. It's always been extremely hard for her living so far away. Travel was costly and time-consuming, and she had a different set of complexities living so far away, as I had living close. She was now doing her best to visit twice a year, and her main objective when coming this time was to organise the finances that Mum was beginning to lose the ability to cope with.

Money was always something Mum had always been extremely capable of managing, and when I broached the subject of her perhaps needing some help with it, she'd always insisted she didn't need help, she had it all sorted. It turns out this wasn't the case any more, and was becoming a worry for everyone involved.

Over the years, she had routinely bought things on credit card to get the points and bonuses, and paid it off every month. It turned out she had somehow stopped doing this several months earlier, in May, either thinking she had already paid it or lost the ability to do so. I'm pretty certain it had become an *'I must go and do that'* which it turned out she didn't go and do. We will never know, but what Ann discovered was a huge unpaid credit card bill and increasing interest.

Mum would have been devastated to know this had happened; she has never missed a payment in her life before, and Ann spent hours on the phone to the credit card company and in the bank to resolve the issue. Shopping online had become tricky anyway, with Mum ordering the same blouse twice, maybe three times. There was a dripping tap of purchases, large and small, which for the last 40 years had been managed to military precision. But in a few short months, it had come home to roost, and the bomb we had suspected had been lying ready, now needed the wires carefully cut to make it safe.

I've heard many stories from others with parents in a similar situation, and the fallout can be devastating. It's a delicate balance of wanting to help without the person feeling they are useless. Just one more thing that's been taken away from them. Much as I had wanted to tackle this job, it was very hard when Mum was totally convinced she was managing. And with working full time, I simply didn't have the time to spend several hours a day for a week sorting it all out.

Thankfully, we had organised the lasting Power of Attorney, which made things easier in a practical sense, but enforcing that power, even when it's to protect a person from themselves, isn't easy at all. It's a painful and emotional process, and although in her 'right mind' Mum would know it was absolutely the best thing to do, in her bewildered dementia mind she didn't always agree or understand. But thankfully, she went along with it.

Ann was in her organised element (she's much better at it than me), working tirelessly to sort everything out, and she was a tower of strength. All the finances were eventually sorted and streamlined, with full instructions for everyone about what went where. When she went back to America, I felt a huge weight of burden had been lifted off my shoulders and I couldn't thank my sister enough for her support and persistence. The relief was enormous.

The day Ann left coincided with a trip to Glasgow for Roy and me. We were visiting my son and, for reasons listed below (taken from my blog post 24 hours after our arrival), the experience speaks for itself.

Summary of the last 24 hours:

Arrived in Glasgow for Status Quo gig (Husband and son going, I would rather eat my own feet), to discover along with several others that they were one year early. ONE YEAR – how the heck did the ticket woman not pick that up when I called her to say we had no tickets yet.

Ate all the food.

Went Christmas shopping, bought a ton of stuff for myself.

Went to the Christmas market and took a ride on the big wheel. Turns out it's powered entirely by my fear, as I was so scared I nearly burst out crying. Husband didn't bat an eyelid. Son held my hand the whole way, telepathically trying to shut me up.

Drank gin to calm nerves.

Went to get my eyebrows threaded (ripped out and tidied up using a piece of cotton thread, true story), and the look of horror on the woman's face made me break the ice by saying, 'Yeah, I know they're in pretty bad shape – this is an emergency.' And she replied, 'Yes, you are right, this is emergency treatment', and it wasn't massively awkward at all.

Went back and did actual Christmas shopping, walked ten million miles, and registered 15 minutes' exercise on my watch. Harsh.

Nearly had an epileptic fit when hubby insisted on telling Alexa to change the light colour in our friend's house like a hundred times.

Haemorrhaged bank account on Christmas shopping and forgot basics like teabags and something for tea.

Downloaded Deliveroo app.

Aside from the fun (!) we had in Glasgow, it was also a learning curve for me and an insight into what life might be like for Mum. After so long in Orkney and away from city life, I was completely de-skilled and void of the ability to perform the basics, or so it felt. There are no trains in Orkney, so when we were coming back from somewhere using busy train stations, crowds were coming at me from all directions. I felt bewildered; I struggled to read the train timetables, and I couldn't work out where we were supposed to be and how to get there.

There was so much stimulation and noise. I was dependent on my son to just tell me what to do and I would follow. I felt like I was a nuisance and useless, too idiotic to manage basic tasks like catching a train. I was so confused I wanted to cry.

As we purchased tickets, I felt proud that this was something I could do. I reached into my purse and grabbed my debit card, holding it up against the machine to do a contactless payment. Nothing happened. So I tried again, with no joy. Then my son gently, kindly, and wordlessly, put his hand over mine and moved down the card until it was pointing at the correct place to make the contactless payment. The machine registered the card and spat the tickets out.

I laughed and thanked him, but for a moment in time I felt first-hand what it must be like for a person with dementia to be fighting this kind of struggle every moment of every waking day. Once again, I inwardly cried. My stone appeared, reminding me it was still there in case I should ever forget, and as we walked back from the station to the house, I saw one solitary flower amidst the cold hard frost. It was pink, with one flower open and two buds bursting with potential. It stood silently despite the frost and -2 degrees air temperature, refusing to give up.

Stooping down to take a photo, I smiled, encouraged that this tiny piece of nature was showing me that we too are all capable of doing hard things, like flowering in winter.

December

'Be near me, Lord Jesus, I ask thee to stay, close by me forever and love me I pray.'
(The daily prayer of my heart)

When I was a little girl, my mother used to sing to me at bedtime. Her repertoire wasn't huge. It was *Wide, Wide as the Ocean*, *All Things Bright and Beautiful*, and *Away in a Manger*. I have such happy memories of this happening, Mum kneeling by the bed and singing. I loved it. Stretching further back to beyond where my memory reaches, I apparently used to request that she sang to me by saying, 'Sing awayning, Mummy, sing awayning.' I don't ever recall not being able to pronounce 'away in' but this memory has been repeated to me many times over the years. Even most recently, Mum still recounts this.

For a long time, I have struggled with Christmas. This dates back to years of single parenting at a season which only served to put a magnifying glass on my aloneness. I know I used to say every year that I just wanted to make it through from December 1st to January 1st relatively unscathed. Attending parties and events alone, watching the children open their presents alone, and opening mine alone, with no real end in sight. I would cry myself to sleep every Christmas night for years.

I don't write this to garner pity or sympathy; I just write it because that was the reality. Childhood Christmases were pretty traditional, but Mum often had to work as a Ward Sister. She firmly believed that she couldn't ask her staff to work shifts that she wasn't prepared to work herself. So, Christmas morning, she would get up and leave early, and we would go in later and have Christmas dinner at the small Birmingham Skin Hospital where she worked. Mum would always arrange for Santa to make one final stop off at the hospital to give us a present. One time, he brought me a silver chain with an S on it.

I believed in Father Christmas for as long as I possibly could, to hold onto the magic. Even now, Christmas Eve is still my favourite time. It holds a sense of magic and anticipation that has never left me. I recall one Christmas Eve visiting my nan, and as I went to the car to go home, I looked up into the sky just in case I got a sighting. I still go out into the night on Christmas Eve and look up into the sky.

This year was a breathtakingly crystal-clear evening with 'stars in the bright sky' and the sound of the sea in the background. I was completely wrung out, at the end of my rope, and full of grief. I'd been feeling close to breaking point, and took the opportunity to enjoy a few minutes of silence as I stood barefoot on the grass, looking up at the sky, just in case. Little did I know that being stretched to my limit was about to go to a whole new level.

★

Despite being vaguely ready for Christmas in terms of having dutifully bought the bulk of the presents, I was nowhere near emotionally ready. Every year it creeps up on me. I become aware of it for months before, as shops insist on their constant round of stocking products continually out of season. Easter Eggs in January, Halloween in July, Christmas in August. We are constantly reminded of the next event coming up, months in advance. There seems to be little 'in the moment' when it comes to shopping, but Christmas starts its warm-up around summertime, I'm sure.

December was a seesaw of mixed emotions. I was emotionally exhausted and run down, but also feeling positive about turning 50. I was bereft at what I imagined to be the last Christmas where my mum would really have much input into what was going on, and I was feeling terribly sentimental – an energy I just couldn't switch off. But I was also feeling positive about an upcoming birthday party, organised at the last minute.

All year, my daughter had been persuading me to do something special for my birthday and at least mark it in some way, and all year I had been avoiding the issue.

I don't like organising parties and don't really cope with them on any kind of grand scale. I have a house that permanently needs work doing to it ,and I struggle to keep on top of, plus 100 other excuses as to why people wouldn't want to come.

Having a birthday that falls slap-bang in the middle of Christmas celebrations also means people would be double-booked and have other commitments far more exciting than mine. I have two lovely friends who I was discussing this with. We were comparing 'introverts: we are all crap at parties' notes, and one of them suggested I have a very simple open house with a bring-and-share buffet. That way, people with other commitments in the afternoon or evening could still come.

It was like a light went on and felt like something I could manage. So, I sent out a save the date in the nick of time, and organised it for mid-December, just a couple of days after my birthday, calling it my '350th in dog years'.

When the see-saw dipped, it was hard. I was desperate to swim and it had been eight days since my last outdoor swim. It felt like everything was conspiring against me to stop me going, which sounds a little dramatic, but when you're a sea swimming addict...

I finally made it into the water on December 3rd in Finstown – a central point between Kirkwall and Stromness. There's a slipway, so entry into the water is easy, but it's very seaweedy so only enjoyable at high tide where you can dodge it. Swimming across to the little pier at the end of someone's garden and back again gives you a decent workout, and for some reason Finstown is always a couple of degrees colder than anywhere else in Orkney. We've theorised as to why, and can only surmise that it gets a lot of run-off from the fields nearby, fresh water being colder and coming across the land. But that's only a theory.

I was a little nervous after a break away from things, if only for a week or so. It's surprising how quickly you lose your nerve, so you have to keep on getting in for the sake of holding your nerve and acclimatisation.

I walked down the slipway and the cold hit me like a brick. It was uncomfortably cold, the heavy breathing kind, and my legs felt like pins and needles. The usual collection of screeching and squealing told me others felt it too, and the water measured five degrees, but acclimatisation quickly kicked in. If I could push past the discomfort, I knew I would be ok, and I managed to swim out to the pier and back again before slipping into warm clothes and having my trusty, unspilled, hot chocolate to hand.

In Orkney, they say you have nine months of terrible weather and then it's winter. In the summer, I would say that was unfair, but as autumn bleeds into winter I always start to say it's a true assessment. We were approaching the longest night and the weather was not favourable for swimming. It wasn't so much the cold as the wind and dark, combined with other commitments, making it difficult.

Several swims were called off due to high winds, and I wasn't swimming anywhere near as much as I had been. I felt it affecting my mood as well as my health. I'd always known it was keeping my mood lifted, but it was only when opportunity went that I realised how down I was becoming. With a bit of effort, I managed a dip in the dark before work once, meeting others to swim, but not always knowing who I was swimming with and not being able to recognise them if I met them in daylight!

We met at Inganess, where an unexploded torpedo had been found a few miles away the previous day. This spooked me more than seals. Even though I had swum near it hundreds of times, I just hadn't known it was there. A local fisherman had brought it in with his catch, and it had been taken out to sea to finally be detonated 'safely'. It was strange to think of the remnants of the evils of war still hanging around. It had lain dormant for nearly 80 years, thankfully never fulfilling the purpose for which it was created: to cause harm to others.

Disappointingly, I wasn't able to manage a last-day-in-my-forties swim because of the awful weather and high winds. But I was determined to swim on my 50th birthday come what may, and ended up double dipping. The first was in my lunch break, where I donned an inflatable crown and swam at Scapa with friends. My husband called me the queen of the sea, and I felt it. Turning 50 had been life-changing, as I reflected back on all that I'd achieved by trying all these new experiences.

On my birthday, I'd already woken and eaten

Maltesers for breakfast, voted in the election, worn a badass crown like a boss to swim in freezing seas, and the day was still young!

My second swim was at Ness, and it was a full moon on a beautiful calm and clear night. The last full moon of the decade, and utterly magical. There is something breathtaking about swimming in moonlight as it hits the water and your surroundings are gently lit. Having only done it twice, it was really memorable to enter a new decade of my life in such a way. A friend came with sparklers, which she bravely tried to light a hundred times with much determination, and friends sang Happy Birthday to me in the water.

Many of my gifts had been sea-themed, including a ring from Mum and Dad in the shape of a wave, a necklace cast from a starfish, a charm bracelet with shell charms from my daughter, and other delights. Friends and family told me I deserved to feel loved, and on my special day I truly did feel loved by so many.

A couple of days later, I held my 350th, and the party I'd been so nervous about hosting ended up being a truly memorable day. Serving mulled wine or warm spiced apple punch for the drivers, people came and stayed and chatted and laughed, and we had the most fun-filled time with friends. I was so pleased I'd been persuaded to hold the party and had a fabulous time.

Fiona had always loved parties, and was famous for her fabulous birthday cakes. For my fortieth, she'd made me an After Eight cake, and was always so creative. Her husband arrived at the party and walked in saying, 'What would Fiona do?' He then produced a cake made in her mixer, and candles on it spelling out the age, 350 in dog years! It was exactly the kind of thing Fiona would have done, and everyone at the party knew it. There was not a dry eye in the house, and it was bittersweet to feel that she was almost there with me for the celebration.

It was a wonderful and relaxed party that went on into the early hours. For a short time, I was able to lay aside my living grief and enjoy the moment without fear of what the future held in terms of Mum and Dad. For a short while the see-saw was up.

December is always a busy month with lots going on, and I had the pleasure of going to another ballet, this time with both Mum and Dad. It was a live streaming of *Copélia* from the Royal Opera House, and both parents were delighted to come, so I was able to meet them from work. I worry about Dad driving on dark, cold, and windy nights, but he was happy to do it and as usual arrived early for our meet-up.

I knew now I was making memories for myself. Capturing every moment and making it all count, as though I could see the sands of time slipping away faster and faster. I was filled with joy for doing these things, and simultaneously filled with regret for not having done more. I know my parents would never want me to feel this way. They have always wanted their children to be independent and live full lives without needing to be attached to them, but I put this down to part of the living grief process I was going through. With grief comes regret and, looking back, I was simply going through that process.

While we waited for the ballet to start, a live streaming of *La Bohème* was advertised for late January – Dad's favourite. I made a mental note to ensure we got to that, too. He was working so hard to care for Mum now and deserved to get to his favourite opera, even if it meant he cried at the end – as he confessed, he always did.

Mum and I also made it along to a charity bingo evening in the community hall close to where she lives. Some people take their bingo very seriously, and woe betide any larking around. But a friend and I go to the occasional fundraising one, try to keep up with the professionals, and enjoy the fixed routine of an Orkney bingo night for a bit of fun. I was telling Mum about having been to one a few months ago, and she said she would have loved to come and asked if I could take her next time.

Worrying she wouldn't keep up, I had been reluctant to take her, but spoke to the others I was going with about her desire to come. In the grand scheme of things, what did it matter if she shouted bingo at the wrong time, or missed shouting and lost a token gift? Did it really matter as long as she had fun? I have no idea why a stupid bingo game consumed me with so much pain, but that Friday before we went it felt like I had cried on and off all day.

I collected Mum and, in the car, spoke about perhaps

sharing a set of books. Mum agreed, saying she thought she would only manage one. I was filled with relief, and as we went in and found our seats, I was so thankful as an army of white-haired ladies in cardigans recognised Mum and showed her such kindness. People said hello to her, and I knew at times she didn't recognise them any more but politely said hello back. Others she did recognize, and spoke away fine to. She enjoyed the evening very much.

There's always a break in the middle when sandwiches and home bakes are served. Mum had no qualms about eating three pieces of cake, and we laughed at an overweight daughter (me!) moderating her slim mother's eating habits. But after an anxious day worrying about how it would all work out, I could go to bed thankful that a charity bingo night had been a huge success in a small and gentle way. My mother could play one bingo book, eat cake, and delight in a raffle prize. She was enjoying the moment and that was all that mattered.

As we were leaving, a woman stopped me and said, 'I don't know you, but I recognised you from the magazine article you wrote. I just want to say you cared for your mum so beautifully this evening, and she's lucky to have you as a daughter.' I wept.

I was working right up until Christmas Eve and was physically and emotionally exhausted. As we approached the longest night, I felt just about on my hands and knees. There's a small psychological shift in me once solstice is over and the days begin to slowly lengthen, but until that point it feels like I'm travelling around in perpetual darkness. Driving to work in the dark, driving home in the dark, and barely any light in the middle of the day.

It's draining, but as Christmas lights begin to appear in windows and gardens, a glimmer of hope sparkles, and I was super excited to have the children home for a few days. This is the hardest thing I find about living in Orkney. I am so far away from my children and miss them terribly. Whilst I want them to have great lives and be fulfilled, there's an emptiness when they aren't here.

The plan was that Katie would travel up to Aberdeen from London by train and meet her brother, before they both got on the Aberdeen boat which brings the students and family home for Christmas. It's always wise to plan this a few days in advance, because there's been times it's been cancelled due to poor weather, and contingency plans need to be made. But thankfully the weather looked to be safe enough for their crossing, and I began to relax a little knowing they would make it over without hitch. However, things began to unravel very quickly, taking me to a new breaking point.

★

We'd recently fitted a new bathroom (seesaw up) and I was at home with a terrible cold (seesaw down). I'm now pretty certain the fact I even caught a cold was because I'd spent so little time in the saltwater this month (seesaw down, down). Belief is that the immune system is strengthened by outdoor swimming, but also that salt stored in the nose from all the sea swimming serves to prevent colds. I haven't researched this hugely, but speaking for myself, I think there's some truth in it.

Along with the new bathroom, we'd acquired some new doors at a good price and a friend was coming over to help Roy fit them. This was a friendly but noisy affair, and I had little time to be ill. Katie was on a train bound for Aberdeen, and Elliot would be joining her the next day. My seesaw was cranking up.

The phone rang and it was Katie crying and distressed to the point of incoherence.

'You're going to have to slow down and calm down, Katie, I can't understand a word you're saying.'

Eventually she managed to get the words out between sobs so that I could understand. Whilst on her train, she'd heard the most awful, dreadful sound and then the train screeched to a halt. All the passengers looked around, wondering what on earth had happened. Katie even commented to another passenger about it, and at one point wondered if part of the train had somehow derailed.

An announcement quickly followed that sadly a passenger had gone in front of the train to end their life. I won't say 'jumped', because I hate the expression. Maybe they just stood there, maybe they walked out in front. Who knows how they came to be so utterly desperate that they came to be in front of a fast-moving train? But it was devastating, and Katie was distraught to have been on the train when it happened.

She cried and cried, and I felt for her aloneness as she waited between carriages to speak to me. I thought of the family left behind to hear the news – something we knew before they did. I thought of the train driver, the emergency services, and the desperate person for whom life was too much.

The whole thing dampened our spirits somewhat, and Katie was unsettled and tearful for days. She eventually made it to her accommodation in Aberdeen and met her brother Elliot for lunch the following day. They sent me a cheeky selfie of them before boarding the boat, and late on Saturday night we made the familiar drive down to the pier to meet them. It was a joyous reunion and I was over the moon to have my babies back in the nest. Things were going to be fine. The seesaw was back up.

The following day, I invited Mum and Dad over for dinner. I'd made roast lamb, everyone's favourite, and the children could get some precious time with their grandparents and vice-versa.

Katie struggled to eat her roast dinner, though, and complained of not feeling great, but initially we put it down to blues from the horrible train incident. We'd managed a big shop earlier in the day and everyone was in high spirits. Christmas was a couple of days away, everything was finally organized, and I was so looking forward to stopping on Christmas Eve and enjoying a well-earned nine daybreak. Mum and Dad would come over on Christmas Day and bring with them a finely cooked turkey, something Mum has done since forever and wasn't about to relinquish this tradition, dementia or no dementia!

We played family games that Sunday night and laughed until we cried. I don't ever remember laughing so hard for so long as I do that evening. Even Elliot, the quiet one, laughed along with us. It was tremendous fun and my grief left me for a while. I just had two more days to get through at work.

On Christmas Eve, before I'd even left the house, I had a phone call from Roy. He often rings to tell me if the roads are bad and to take care, and I assumed it was that. But he was ringing to say his car was in the ditch and he was just waiting for someone to come and pull him out. He'd come off the road in the ice, and ironically the gritter was the first vehicle to stop. He was fine and unhurt, but the car had been damaged and a tyre was punctured. He was working all over Christmas, and everywhere would be closed. We were thankful he was unhurt, but it couldn't have come at a worse time.

I left work on Christmas Eve feeling exhausted and so ready for a break. Katie loves cooking and was going to do the Christmas dinner, and I was looking forward to a restful few days ahead, doing jigsaw puzzles and eating Quality Street for breakfast, whilst simultaneously complaining I was fat. The usual festive stuff awaited.

Our traditional Christmas Eve supper was planned

and executed, but Katie ate very little. Our usual carol service attendance didn't happen as we were all too tired, so we watched a Christmas movie and Katie went to bed feeling unwell. Despite everything feeling a little flat, I still took the time to stand outside and look up for the magic of Christmas Eve, and had a few minutes of contemplation before being the last one to go to bed.

I was woken in the early hours by Katie, who was becoming more unwell. She now had diarrhoea and terrible cramping in her stomach, and we rang NHS 24. We were advised it was a virus and to self-medicate with Imodium and stay in bed. (On reflection, it was probably the worst advice, but we could only work on hindsight.) By the following morning, Katie looked and felt terrible and was too unwell to join us for Christmas dinner.

Mum and Dad came over, I cooked, and forgot half the things, but no-one really noticed. We had a nice meal but felt sorry for Katie. All my worries about Mum had come to nothing, as she'd been fine, but it was a mish-mash of a day and had not been terribly restful. Katie didn't really surface the entire day and we all went to bed feeling rather flat but slightly relieved it was all over. I'd even managed a fun Christmas Day dip with the Polar Bears and swum in Santa hats, which had been a joyous hour.

It had been a mixed day, rather like life was feeling at the moment, but in the early hours Katie text me from the bathroom. *Mum, please take me to hospital. I'm in so much pain.* It was absolutely chilling.

What I could do at this point is give a taxi driver rant now about the stupidity of the NHS 24 system. Hours of ringing, explaining symptoms, waiting for someone to ring back, waiting for another someone to ring back to be told she needs to be seen and take her to hospital, which was information I could have told them hours before. Rage! I could, but I won't.

I eventually got her in the car to drive the 18 miles to hospital, whilst stopping off at public toilets on the way. The pain was becoming unbearable for her, and she recalls it as the worst journey of her life. Should I have called an ambulance? Possibly, but I had wanted to leave it for someone who may need the facilities more, if we could manage.

Katie was assessed and moved to a ward, where she remained for six days severely ill. She had CT scans and a colonoscopy, which couldn't be fully completed as her bowel was so inflamed and ulcerated. She was only allowed home on New Year's Eve because she managed to persuade the doctors she would be looked after by me and would return if she should worsen. It turned out she had severe campylobacter, which is food poisoning from the chicken she ate in the restaurant in Aberdeen, but there were also worrying symptoms indicating Crohn's disease or ulcerative colitis.

She was very unwell, and I'd spent the Twixmas holiday driving to and from the hospital, sleeping in hospital chairs, washing nighties, and holding sick bowls. (Twixmas is a thing; it's the bit between Christmas and New Year where we all fall down a black hole of eating and not knowing what day it is – a bit like quarantine life!)

My seesaw dipped, crash landed, and completely fell over. There was no way up. I had reached rock bottom and couldn't climb out. I hated seeing my daughter in so much pain and distress; I hated causing Mum and Dad more worry, as I knew they would; and I was so, so, so tired.

New Year's Eve plans were cancelled. We were all worried about Katie, and I felt stretched so thin and pulled in so many different directions that I didn't know what to do with myself. I felt completely and utterly broken and had absolutely nothing left. I was writing a book about how sea swimming helped me cope with what life chucks at us, and on the last page of the final chapter I couldn't cope. I felt like I was a fraud, an imposter, and a fake. Life well and truly sucked, and I had flatlined.

On the last day of the decade I went to my GP and dissolved into tears. My doctor was very compassionate and understanding, and helped me to see that from the outside looking in I'd had more than my fair share of life stresses to deal with. I was signed off work for a few weeks, and this brought me some breathing space and a chance to get the much-needed rest I'd been yearning. But it reinforced my feelings of failure. Lack of sleep, stress and exhaustion, all took its toll. I wanted to sleep for five years, hit the snooze button, and sleep for another five. Stick a fork in me, guys, I'm done.

Sing awayning, Mummy – sing awayning.

January 2020

I used to belong to a book group, which gradually faded when we spoke less about the book and more about the wine we were drinking. But at the time, I was often jibed for choosing books that didn't have a neat and tidy happy ending. My argument was always that it was totally unrealistic to expect such a thing. Life isn't like that, and it has shown me this time and time again. The boy doesn't always get the girl; they don't always live happily ever after; friends die despite our fervent prayers; we don't find a winning lottery ticket; it rains and we all get wet; undeserving people get dementia and become bewildered; their children cry in cars.

As January yawned into life, I didn't wake with a new year, new me attitude. Realistically, it was harder than ever, and the crying continued. Katie slowly recovered enough to return to her life and work in London, where she is receiving ongoing tests, diagnosis, and treatment for her illness.

In absolute desperation for some solitude and respite, I found an Airbnb in the Highlands and booked myself a couple of nights away, oscillating between urgently needing a break and a rest, feeling full of anxiety and guilt about leaving Mum and Dad, and feeling like I 'should' be doing, doing, doing but not having the energy or motivation to do anything. I went with their blessing, and had some blissful days of rest and solitude.

The B&B was owned by a lovely couple who intuitively knew what I needed and allowed me to sleep and retreat, emerging only for an evening meal and breakfast. Two nights ended up being four, as I travelled down early to avoid high winds, and travelled back late as the boat was cancelled for the same reason.

Normally I would do anything to avoid travelling on the boat in high winds for fear of being terribly seasick, it's so ghastly. But my determination for solitude made me swallow sea sickness tablets, put on wrist bands, and lie down. We pitched and rolled on the high, stormy seas, but I was absolutely fine. It ended up being a memorable and wonderful few days of solitude and rest, and something I plan to work into my diary in the future on a regular basis.

My mum has lived through an enormous amount of pain and ill health. She's shouldered so much and has demonstrated time and time again that when life knocks you over, you get back up again. It's not easy, but she's shown me on many occasions that it's possible.

I was devastated to hear from Dad that she had asked

the question, 'Has Simon died?' Simon, her son who had died in the most devastating of circumstances eleven years previously, when Mum and Dad had shouldered a whole new level of pain and got back up again. But now, mum was unsure. The haze had come over her memory, the ugly evil dementia had side-swiped us all again, and I was both bereft and furious. Not furious at Mum. I was bereft for the sadness of it all, but I was furious at dementia and made fresh resolve to keep getting back up again and punching it in the face.

On the anniversary of my first time in the water, I met with a group of friends at our local place and the tide was high. Standing on the water's edge, I reflected on the journey I'd been on over the past year and contemplated the road still to be travelled, ever grateful for the enormous blue spaces to escape to in Orkney.

I braced myself for the inevitable breath-taking cold, thanking my heart for saying yes every time my head said no. Walking further into the waves, I took the familiar deep breath, let out a squeal as I put my shoulders under, and began to swim. Once again, I was restored. I was alive and invigorated. Soon there would be snowdrops, and I would do my annual search for them with the promise of hope in the midst of deep winter.

Life is a continuing journey, with a never-ending road of ups and downs. We don't get to write our own endings; we don't know how it's going to work out. We thankfully have no idea what's around the corner; we can only deal with the here and now.

I had difficult challenges ahead, and if I let it, I felt as though life could drown me. Once again, it was sink or swim time.

But I choose to swim.

I choose to swim.

I choose to swim.

Acknowledgements

SOUNDS OSCAR SPEECH KLAXON I might as well acknowledge the elephant in the room. I have so many people to thank who have been directly or indirectly involved in this book that it's going to end up being a gushing speech of emotion worthy of its own red-carpet event. But I really am supremely grateful to so many people, and I don't want to miss anyone. So, strap yourselves in and get ready.

My heartfelt thanks go to…

Cassie, my book mentor, who took my lifetime dream and made it a reality. I've always enjoyed writing and have spent my life saying 'I want to write a book', but never actually getting around to doing so. Thank you, Cassie, for guiding me through the process and drying my tears multiple times. You're like a doula for writers.

Christine, my editor, thank you so much for turning a horror show of grammar errors and typos into something far better. My readers thank you, too; I know this.

Jessica, for taking my terrible sketches and comments – such as *could you make the lighthouse look less like a penis?* – and turning it into a cover image I love. And to Jen, for all your advice and expertise to make the final book cover magic happen. To see it come to life is an enormous joy.

On the subject of magic, thanks to Dave for managing to get the loveliest author photo of me, despite my not having had a haircut for months because of lockdown, and doing it on an incredibly windy beach at a social distance of 2m. How you managed to turn my scary neutral face into someone looking friendly and approachable is nothing short of a miracle. I'm wondering if you could follow me around all the time now, please? It's been a long time in lockdown and things are gettin' ugly round here!

I've been writing a blog for some time now, and I am so grateful to the people who have subscribed and followed via my blog site, Twitter, or Facebook page. Without your encouragement and support, my words just go into the abyss. So, know that if you've taken the time to click a 'like' or sent a comment, it really helps affirm insecure writers and calm the voice of imposter syndrome.

The same goes to the incredible community on Instagram, who message me and chat via DM, stories, and comments on my pictures. Your constant enthusiasm as I banged on about this book helped me to keep going, and gave me the confidence to go ahead and reach the finish line. If you've been part of sharing the love, however small, then know I appreciate you very much. You're all amazing. Now go and do hard things.

To the readers of the manuscript – Amy, Lisa B, Lisa I, Mim, Shauna, and Rachael. Sending out your manuscript is terrifying, as some of you know. I likened it to putting your baby into a bonny baby competition and then coming last because your offspring is actually not that cute. So, thank you enormously for your enthusiasm, help, and feedback about the book.

I am extremely lucky to be surrounded by a huge number of kind and supportive friends, both near and far; some I've never met in real life. If you've listened to my ramblings over the last 12 months, then consider yourselves well and truly thanked. Lynn, Mary, Ingrid, and Hazel – you have dried my tears more than you'll ever know.

I've had a great year swimming, and it all started with the Orkney Polar Bears. Thank you for showing me the ropes and sharing the water (and many cookies!) with me.

My husband, Orkney Beef – I know you don't go in for all this mush, but you know how important writing this book was to me. Thank you for giving me the freedom to follow my dream. You're the kindest man I know.

To my two children, Katie and Elliot. Thank you for reading the manuscript, Katie; and for all your technical help Elliot, and for stepping in when I had an epic meltdown one sunny afternoon. *'All I get is flowers!'* (private joke). But most of all, thanks to both of you for demonstrating such maturity and empathy in the face of so much over the years. You have turned out to be marvellous human beings, and I'm enormously proud of who you both are.

Lastly, to Mum and Dad, the two bravest people I know. Thank you for allowing me to share your story so we can be of help to others facing the same. I love you, and I hope I've made you proud.

Contact Sarah

Author website www.sarahkennedynorquoy.com

Blog www.norqfromork.com

Instagram @seasaltandsarah

Facebook Norq from Ork an Orkney Writer

Twitter @sarahknorquoy

For all enquiries please email

info@sarahkennedynorquoy.com

About the Author

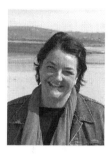

Sarah moved from Cambridge, England, to the Orkney Islands with her two children in 2008 where she now lives with her second husband and dog, Hope. She is often described as hilariously funny, honest and relatable. 'A sheer drop of positivity and happiness'.

When she's not doing her day job as a support worker, you will probably find her swimming in the sea or dreaming about it. She loves writing and shares her observations on life in a funny, sensitive, and self-aware way through her blog and Instagram stories.

Sarah describes herself as an extroverted-introvert, with a love of solitude, a deep passion for finding joy in the every day, and a love of scouring the beaches for tiny pieces of sea glass and pottery washed up on the shore.

Printed in Great Britain
by Amazon